3

Fit Self-Improvement Series

LEGS & THIGHS

3

Fit Self-Improvement Series

LEGS & THIGHS

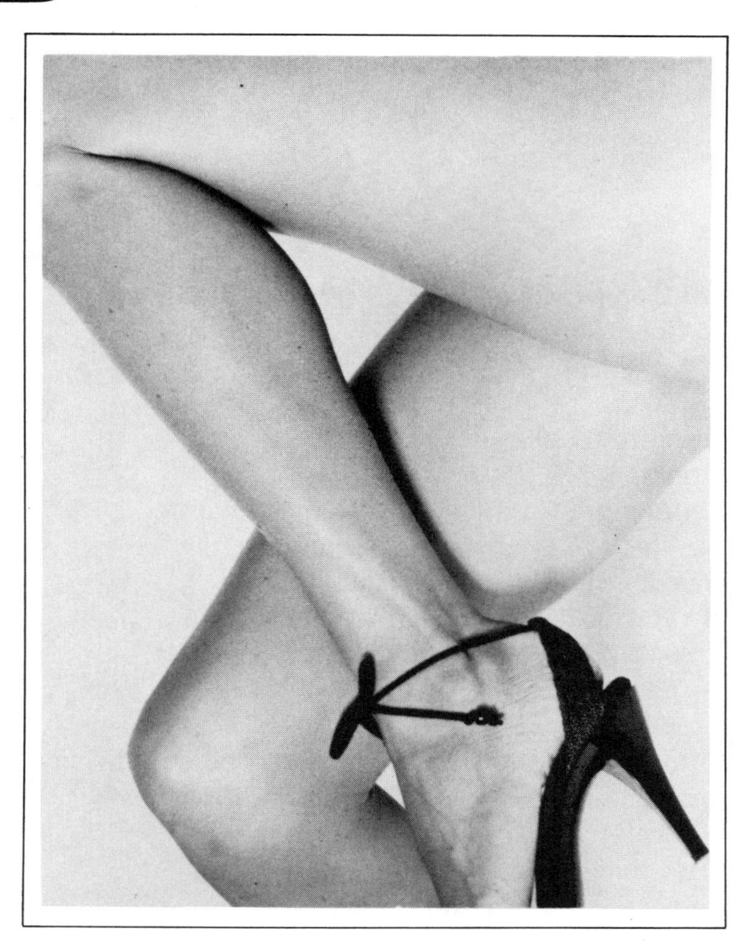

by Cheri Rae Wolpert

and the editors of FiT

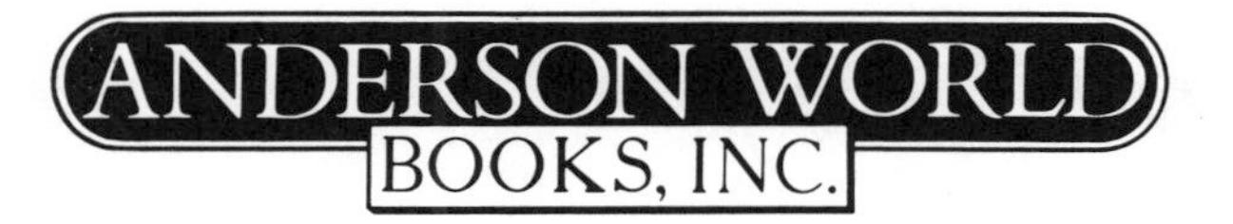

Library of Congress Cataloging in Publication Data
Wolpert, Cheri Rae, 1953—
Legs & thighs.

(Fit self-improvement series; 3)
Bibliography: p. 95
1. Reducing exercises. 2. Exercise for women.
3. Leg. 4. Thigh. 5. Women — Nutrition.
I. Fit magazine. II. Title. III. Series.
RA781.6.W64 1983 613.7'1 83-6371
ISBN 0-89037-260-8

Anderson World Books, Inc.
1400 Stierlin Road
Mountain View, CA
94043

CONTENTS

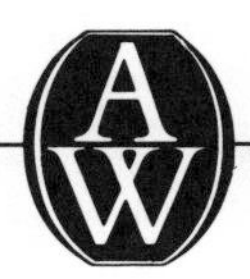

INTRODUCTION

Legs need more than liberal applications of lotions and potions to become beautiful. In order to have strong, sleek legs, you just can't get around the need for exercise. But the instant someone mentions exercise, what negative image pops into your mind? Is it one reminiscent of the boring exercise routines you were forced to do in high school? Remember those ridiculous bloomers and ugly T-shirts that we were required to wear? No wonder so many women associate exercise with unpleasant memories.

Well, times have certainly changed! And luckily, they've definitely changed for the better. The women's liberation movement has changed our perceptions forever. One of the first women to run in the Boston Marathon, Kathrine Switzer, (in 1967) is today a leading figure with Avon Products, and now actively promotes women's sports. And even then, she registered as K. Switzer and bundled up in a dingey sweatsuit to hide the fact that she was a female. We truly have come a long way, baby! Finally, after political pressure from runners around the world, the 1984 Olympics will feature the first women's marathon — the 26.2-mile event. It will say to the world that women are every bit as durable as men.

The prospect of beginning a regular exercise program can seem intimidating. You might think it means long hours of drudgery. But it doesn't. And you can pursue your personal interests. It doesn't matter what sport you take up, as long as it's aerobic and as long as you participate in it four to five times per week for a minimum of fifteen minutes. This level of exercise will maintain good health. If you're trying, after a long period of sedentary living, to become fit, you should work up to a higher level of fitness gradually. The body is incredibly adaptive, and is capable of much more than we regularly demand of it.

The first step in getting started with your shape-up program for lovelier legs and thighs is to buy a notebook to record improvements. Let it be your fitness diary. Treat yourself to an especially nice notebook so that you'll be sure to use it — maybe one with a fabric cover, or leather binding. What do you write in this notebook? Anything you want, but many people find that it's very helpful to keep a record of everything they eat while on a special fitness/diet program. The theory is that if you have to write it down, you might be less likely to overeat, or to eat something that you know is an empty-calorie treat with little nutritional value.

What can you write about besides food in your fitness notebook? How about personal feelings as you see yourself coming closer to your goals? Your new-found confidence as you see your body changing because you're suddenly in charge? The pleasure that you feel because your discipline and commitment to excellence is producing results? All your comments probably won't be quite so rosy, of course. There may be days when you feel completely unattractive, much too heavy, and have nothing good to write about yourself. It's on those down days that you'll really need to refer back to your up days and remember just how good you can feel. Recording your thoughts and feelings is an activity that requires some discipline at first. It shouldn't, however, be something that you force yourself to do. Just try to remember to write something daily about your new-found fitness program, and how good you feel about the changes you're making in your life.

Another important use for your notebook is as a place to keep all those photos from fitness, fashion and sports magazines that motivate and inspire you. You know, the ones that show beautiful, fit young women wearing clingy dresses, skimpy shorts, the barest bikinis and the trimmest jeans. Cut them out and paste them down in your notebook so that you can focus on the makings of beautiful, fit women. Pay special attention to those women that you most admire; notice that they aren't cookie-cutter look-alikes. Fit women are no different from all women — they come in various shapes and sizes.

Think of a few women who figure prominently in the world of endurance sports: Julie Leach, who won the October 1982 Ironman triathlon; Gayle Olinekova, about whom *Sports Illustrated* said, "the greatest legs to ever stride the earth"; Billie Jean King, who paved the way for the multi-millionaire tennis players today; Chris Evert-Lloyd, Tracy Austin and Martina Navratilova. These women are in great shape, from the ground up.

If you're a fan of old movies and memorabilia, you'll surely remember that Betty Grable's gorgeous gams were insured for a half-million dollars; film star of the forties, Leslie Brooks, won the Hosiery Designer of America's award for best legs, with the measurements of ankle eight inches, calf fourteen inches, thigh twenty and a half inches; and who could ever forget the classic Marilyn Monroe shot in the movie *"The Seven Year Itch"* with her skirt lifted by a draft of air to reveal her shapely legs?

Film stars of the past certainly have no monopoly on beautiful legs. Consider the incredible talent and strength of dancers like Juliet Prowse and Cyd Charisse. Remember the suggestive scene with Anne Bancroft in *"The Graduate,"* her wonderful legs and black stockings bringing new meaning to Dustin Hoffman's life? Or the long, well-built legs used in the promotion of *"For Your Eyes Only"*? *"10"* star, Bo Derek, who gave an entirely new meaning to Ravel's *Bolero,* said in a recent magazine article that she favors her calves over any other part of her body. Clearly, beautiful, long legs keep us going, keep us glowing and move us right along.

Speaking of moving along, let's do just that as we explore the world of legs and thighs. As one ad promotion says, "Nothing beats a great pair of legs."

1 GETTING STARTED

The journey of a thousand miles begins with a single step.

—Lao-Tse

Congratulations! You're reading this book because you're interested in your body — how it looks, functions and feels. You must have an awareness of your overall health and fitness, and you're determined to maintain and perhaps increase it. You've made a commitment to learn all you can to reach your potential because you care enough about yourself to make the most of what you are. Pursuing fitness is like giving yourself a pat on the back.

Okay, now it's time to have some fun. First, think about your body and how you see yourself. Do you stride purposefully through your daily life? Are your movements strong, comfortable and confident? Do you face new and unfamiliar situations with a smile? Or do you shuffle through your daily life, taking baby steps and worrying about your every move? When people see you, do they automatically think of you as a winner? Or do you project something else? Now think about how first impressions are lasting ones. How do you want to project yourself to the rest of the world? Is it consistent with the real you or is it a little different? Or even a lot different? Well, the good news is that you have a choice; however you want to look, it's up to you.

What I just wrote is not entirely true; there are physical characteristics given us by heredity. You may have inherited your mother's thick ankles or your father's muscular calves. So if you want reed-thin legs, you're going to spend a lifetime wishing for something that's just not possible. When you take stock of your legs, realize what's possible and what isn't. Don't strive to look like someone else who has inherited characteristics that society sees as better — slim, shapely legs. Instead, celebrate your uniqueness. No two pair of legs are shaped the same. Your goal is to never give up reaching for your potential.

RELAXATION TECHNIQUE

Your first step is to visualize how you actually look. Find a comfortable place where you can relax and concentrate. Take the phone off the hook, dim the lights and turn off the radio. Now, sitting on the floor, slowly begin to relax your entire body, starting with your toes, then your calves and your thighs. Let the day's tensions melt away as you relax your body, one part at a time. Now relax your fingers, your arms, your abdomen, your chest and your shoulders. Pay particular attention to your shoulders and your neck; many of us carry a great deal of tension here. Relax the muscles in your face and your scalp; feel your body without tension, in a state of total relaxation. Doesn't that feel good? Whenever the demands of your day get to you, if you do this relaxation exercise it will help you immeasurably.

Now that your whole body is relaxed, it's time to be aware of your body. Clear away all the clutter of the day and focus on your body. What do you see? Is it easy for you to visualize how you really look, from the ground up? Or do you find yourself only able to focus on one particular part of your body? Maybe it's your face, your hair or your body from the waist up. It's important not to be judgmental during this exercise. Just be observant of your feelings and your reactions as you proceed. Once you bring your entire body into focus, change your focus so that you are more aware of your legs. Are you visualizing yourself naked or clothed?

Pay attention to all the details. If you're seeing yourself clothed, notice the type of clothing, how it fits and how comfortable it feels on you. If you're naked, notice the texture of your skin, the muscle definition in your thighs and your calves. Notice the hair on your legs, the bruise or two you may have, any scars, broken veins or areas of cellulite that may be part of your legs. No cringing or wincing allowed here; we're just visualizing our bodies objectively — remember, don't make any judgments about how you look.

When you've visualized your legs entirely, front and back, visualize how they feel to you. Are they strong and muscular or are they flabby and weak? Maybe you think that they are thin, or even skinny. Just be aware of how you see your legs in your mind's eye. Focus on that image and keep it there. It may be helpful for you to take the time to make a few notes in your fitness notebook so that you can refer back to this exercise. Now, describe the legs that you visualized as yours.

Now for a little reality checking; open your eyes and look at your legs in a full-length mirror. Again, wincing is not allowed. Just observe your legs and thighs as though you're just seeing them for the first time. This might just be the first time that you're taking an objective look at this part of your body. Notice all the details, the unique shape, maybe the funny little scar on your knee, or your smooth shins, your strong quadriceps. Now, while you're observing your legs, jot down just how they look to you, noting both good and not-so-good points. In your fitness notebook, write down as accurately as you can how your legs look to you.

The next part of our little exercise is the most fun. It's time for you to use your imagination and just let yourself go. Turn off all the voices inside your head, put on some soothing music and let your creative powers be fully expressed. Imagine how you would like to look. Notice your expressions, your body carriage, your walk, your clothing. Do you have that image well focused in your mind? Great. Now we're going to be a little more specific, so make sure that you see yourself just the way you want. Don't be afraid to adjust here and there. This is your opportunity to create the body that you've always wanted. Get it the way you want it, right down to the last detail — imagine your fingernails, your hairstyle, your waist, your ideal hips, thighs and calves.

Once you've got your body in focus, narrow your vision to include just your lower half. Visualize your legs problem-free, without a trace of cellulite, bumps or bruises. See them as soft, smooth, tanned and strong, as you would like for them to be. Put that picture in your mind and keep it there so that you will always remember it. Now back to reality; grab your pen and notebook once again and describe in great detail your ideal body, especially your ideal legs and thighs. Doesn't that feel good?

You may be wondering just what was the purpose of these three exercises. Have you heard the old expression of mind over matter? We just gave you an opportunity to unleash the powers of your mind in order to create the you that you want to become. In the first exercise, we permitted you to focus on all those flaws that you imagine in your mind. Chances are you imagine your body somewhat differently than you really appear. That's why we had you do some reality checking in front of the full-length mirror. It's important for you to know whether you're being too harsh or too lenient on yourself. All of us have had the opportunity to tell a friend how nice she looks, and have her answer, "Are you kidding? I need to lose ten pounds!" As you may very well know, each individual's perceptions may change the reality she perceives to be true. Looking at your body in the mirror can have a profound effect if you will be receptive to the experience. Finally, the third exercise allowed you to create, possibly for the first time in your life, your ideal body in fine detail.

FINDING MOTIVATION

Before you take off on your self-improvement journey, in order to create the legs and thighs that you really want, it's important to do just a little advance preparation. The more you assess yourself, the better the results you'll achieve. And it's important to have concise, clear goals when you're attempting a change. It's not enough to say, "Oh, I wish I were in better shape." You're far more likely to successfully change your shape if you conduct a detailed analysis of exactly what you want to change.

Think again now of those ideal legs that you created in your mind's eye. Pretty terrific, weren't they? Just what is it that's keeping you from having legs like that? Put a little work into this self-assessment — it will be worth it. Do you eat too much and not exercise enough? Do you find that you would rather sit around at night and watch television instead of exercising? Is it easier for you to sit on the sidelines of life rather than take your place on center stage? Think seriously about this and figure out what it is that has kept you from achieving the results that you want.

The key principle here is knowing what you want. We have all been so programmed in our daily lives to please others, we often ignore the inner voices that really need to be heard. Ignoring and denying these basic wants often leads to frustration, anger and resentment. Each of these unexpressed feelings can be turned inward, sometimes with self-destructive consequences. Going on a binge, depression, that paralyzed feeling of being too tired to do anything but fall into a chair and watch television — all these behaviors are indicative of hidden problems that may keep you from reaching your physical and psychological potential. If you think that your unexpressed feelings may be causing severe problems, therapy may be in order. There are a number of excellent books that may help you take charge of your life if you are having minor doubts. A partial listing follows:

Twelve Inspirational/Self-Help Books

TITLE	AUTHOR	PUBLISHER
The Art of Loving	Erich Fromm	Bantam Books
Being Fat Has Nothing to do with Food	Pat terHeun	Celestial Arts
Born to Win	Muriel James and Dorothy Jongeward	Addison-Wesley
Fat is a Feminist Issue I & II	Susie Orbach	Berkeley Books
I'm OK — You're OK	Thomas A. Harris, M.D.	Avon Books
Jonathan Livingston Seagull	Richard Bach	Avon Books
The Little Prince	Antoine de Saint Exupery	Harcourt, Brace & World, Inc.
Love	Leo Buscaglia	Fawcett Crest
Passages	Gail Sheehy	Bantam Books
The Prophet	Kahlil Gibran	Knopf Books
Psycho-Cybernetics	Maxwell Maltz, M.D.	F.I.C.S., Wilshire Books
What Took You So Long?	Sheldon Kopp	Science and Behavior Books, Inc.

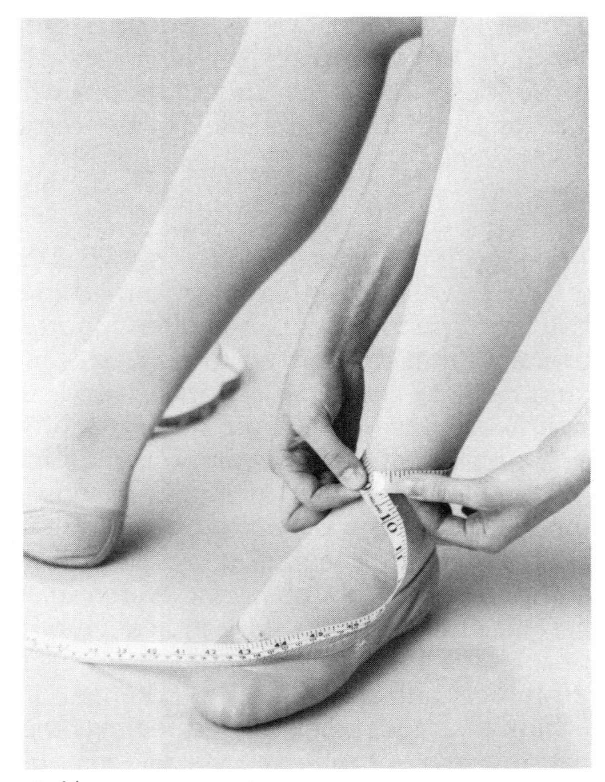

Ankle measurement.

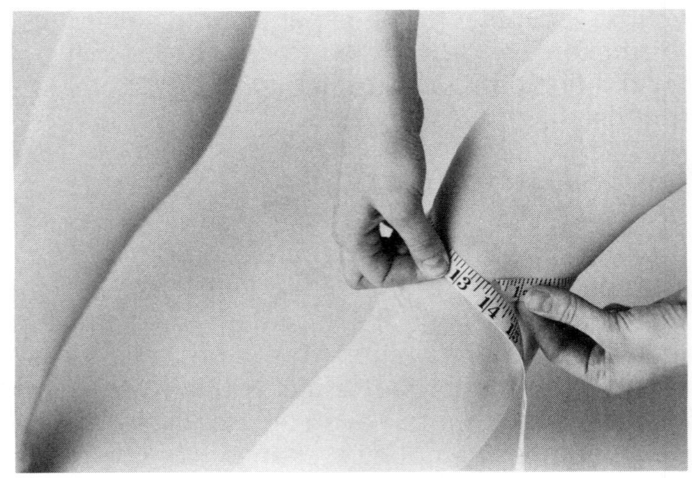

Knee measurement.

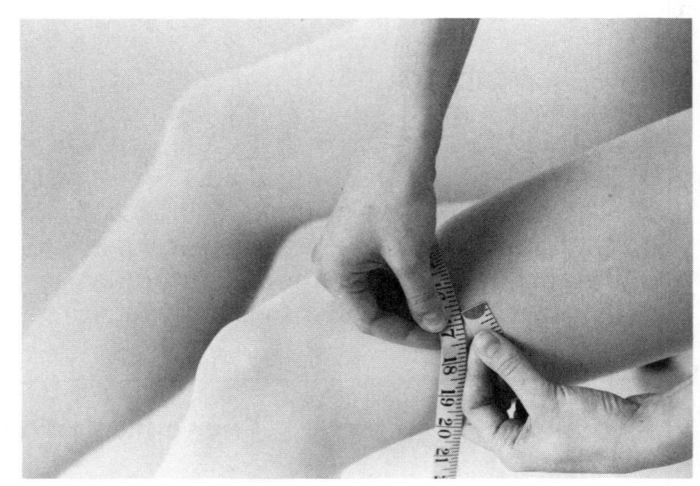

Mid-Thigh measurement.

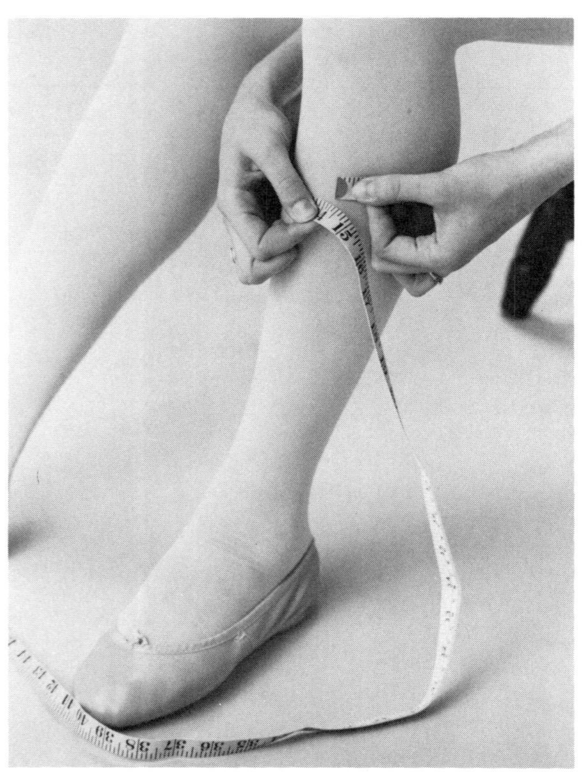

Calf measurement.

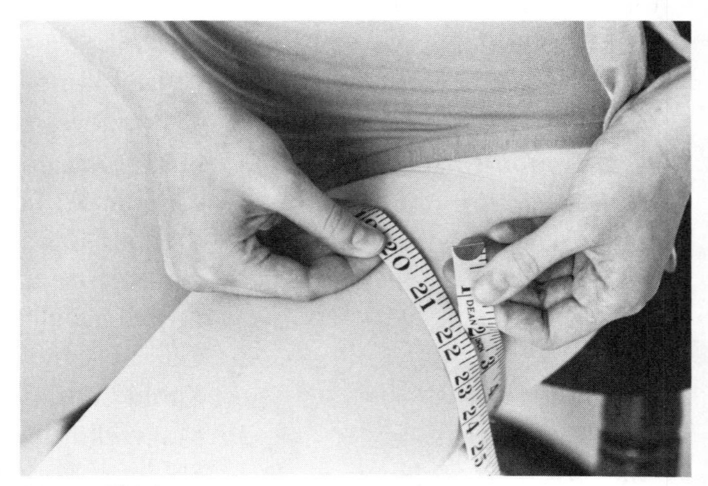

Upper-Thigh measurement.

RIGHT	LEFT	DATE	DATE	DATE	DATE
ANKLES					
CALVES					
KNEES					
MID THIGHS					
UPPER THIGHS					
SPECIAL COMMENTS:					
WEIGHT:					

The point of this is to reiterate what you've heard thousands of times before — each day is a new beginning. e.e. cummings said it best when he wrote:

> *"i thank You God for most this amazing day: for the leaping greenly spirits of trees and a blue true dream of sky; and for everything*
> *which is natural which is infinite which is yes . . . (now the ears of my ears awake and now the eyes of my eyes are opened)*

And now that your ears and eyes are awakened, it's time to go to work and make the changes in your life that will allow you to create those wonderful, beautiful legs you imagined.

GREAT LEGS: HOW TO GET THEM

Commitment is what it takes. You already know exactly what you want; the real trick now is to get started. Since it's a day-to-day proposition, you always have another chance to stay committed to your shape-up program. One way to keep this idea in your mind is to use a little catch phrase that has always served me well:

Personal
Responsibility
In
Daily
Effort

PRIDE — isn't that what it's all about? Once you recognize the powerful feeling that can be derived from taking pride in your appearance and responsibility for making it what you want, you're home free. There's really no secret. The toughest part is getting started — so let's do it.

Take Measure of Yourself

First things first. Put on a leotard and tights or a pair of shorts and a T-shirt. Get out your tape measure so that you can keep an accurate record of your progress. Use the space provided and record measurements of your ankles, calves, knees, mid-thigh and upper thighs. No cheating allowed — this is private information so nobody needs to know it.

It's important that you give yourself plenty of time when you chart your progress. There's nothing more discouraging than being on a program and feeling like it just isn't working. You're not going to see any major changes overnight, but within as little as three weeks, your thighs might look firmer, your clothes might fit differently and you should notice that you have more pep than previously. As we've said, it's important to take this program one day at a time — just remind yourself it took a while for you to get out of shape, and it will be a while before you get back in shape, too. Be patient with yourself and one day, when you're walking down the street, you'll gaze into a shop window and see that the woman with the strong, firm legs is none other than yourself.

2 LOTIONS AND POTIONS

Why should beauty be suspect?

— *Auguste Renoir*

I know you want legs like those beautiful, silky-smooth ones that you see pictured on the cover. Don't we all? But it takes more than exercise, although if you're exercising, you're already halfway there. When you're on the move, you're building beauty from the inside out. Now we're going to learn about what you can do to condition your skin, from the outside in.

Alluring legs that are smooth, well moisturized and free of bumps and dry skin are surprisingly easy to achieve. All it takes is determination and a trip to the nearest drugstore. Stop by any cosmetic counter and you'll find a wide array of tantalizing products that will add to your attractiveness and, ultimately, if one is to believe the product advertisements, your sex appeal.

What are some of these products? To name a few: Depilatories, waxes and beautifully designed shavers give you options in hair removal; lotions, creams and perfumed balms keep your legs soft, smooth and sweet-smelling; tanning lotions have chemicals that can reduce sun damage to your skin, and the supply of sponges, sloughers and special massagers boggles the mind.

IN THE SHOWER

Chances are that as an active woman you spend nearly an hour a day in the shower! That's a fair amount of time, so you ought to learn to make the best of it. Stock your shower with products that can soothe and refresh, invigorate and encourage those tired muscles of yours. After working out so hard, you deserve to indulge a bit — and it's inexpensive and luxurious to try lathers, loofahs, scented soaps and fluffy towels to make your shower time a real pleasure you can look forward to after a tough day.

The first item to consider purchasing is a high-pressure shower head. Marketed under various names, these adjustable, mechanical marvels can be the next best thing to a real massage. Look for one with variable speeds and a pulsating flow for the most versatility. Plan to spend between $15 and $50.

Liquid soaps are very practical in the bath, and they're now available in many scents and colors to suit your pleasure. Some are specially formulated for the sports-minded woman. Bonne Bell's Good Nature Shower 2000 and Vitabath's classic Spring Green scented products are two to try. Both offer nose-tickling herbal scents that may be invigorating after play time. Of course, bar soaps are also acceptable;

just choose one that is fairly mild, like Dove or Ivory. Since you're spending a lot of time coming clean, you don't want to dry your skin with harsh detergent soaps.

When you're bathing, wash your legs with firm, even, long strokes. The slippery feel from the soap and water provides you with a suitable surface during self-massage. Do whatever feels best, but concentrate on kneading sore muscles. Use your knuckles against your thighs for deep massage; use your fingers very lightly over your knees, and use short, deep strokes on your calf muscles. Experiment.

While you're in the shower, find any bumps, bruises or dry, patchy spots you may have developed, and make a note to yourself to correct them. The shower is also a very good place for you to use a loofah or natural sponge to slough off dry skin and to stimulate the circulation in your legs. Rub gently, especially when using a loofah; the secret is to rub, not scrub. You'll notice that after repeated use of an abrasive product, your skin will be softer and smoother. You'll also feel invigorated.

BODY BEAUTIFIERS

Lotions are available in every imaginable fragrance, texture and color. The ingredients, which by law must be listed on the package, may include natural substances like sesame oil, avocado oil, allantoin and cocoa butter, all of which are effective moisturizing agents. Other natural substances that you might try include jojoba and aloe vera extracts. The oils and gels of these plants are becoming more popular as people discover their value.

If you're particular about matching fragrances, try a lotion that matches your favorite perfume or cologne; the added layer of fragrance complements your daily application of spray-on scents.

In choosing a particular lotion for dry skin, the label can't tell you it will work for you. It's the application of that lotion that will really tell. A very good, all-purpose lotion that has become popular in recent years is Vaseline Intensive Care. It is available in both regular and

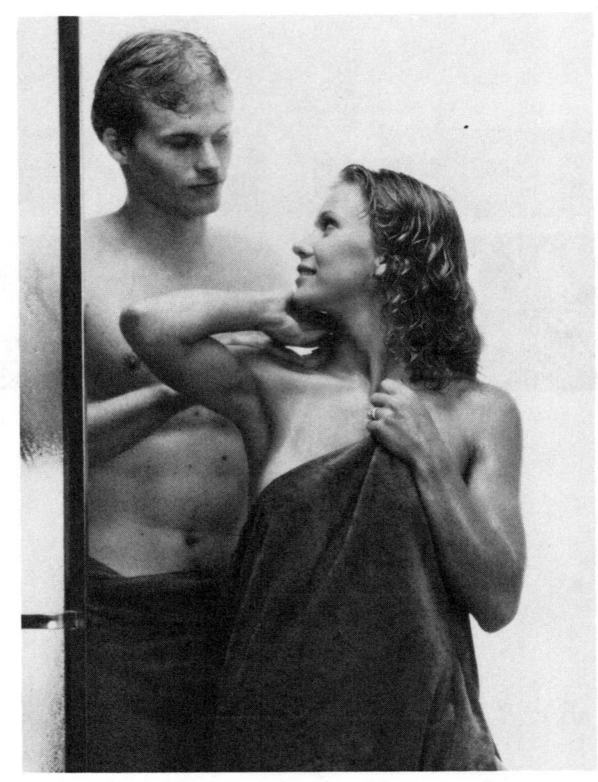

Make your shower an enjoyable part of your day.

herbal scents, and in regular- and extra-strength formulas for extra-dry or damaged skin. This non-sticky, light lotion is effective in moisturizing your dry skin.

The best time to apply lotions or creams to your legs is right after your daily bath or shower. The emollients in the lotions are most effective when the skin is moist, not dry. Towel yourself dry, then apply the lotion. It feels and smells great — if yours doesn't, switch to another brand.

Body Splashes and Toners. There's something delightfully invigorating about body splashes, those scented potions that you literally splash all over your body. They feel particularly good after you've taken a hot shower following a particularly intense workout. Splashes have alcohol and water as their primary ingredients — and the alcohol in the potion leaves you feeling recharged after it evaporates, and it has a nice light scent. When using these products, remember that alcohol dries the skin, so be sure to use plenty of moisturizing lotion afterward. Jean Nate makes an especially popular line of body splash, lotion and powder guaranteed not to clash with your favorite fragrance.

Powder. After you've applied your body splash or lotion, a liberal application of powder is just what you need to provide a smooth finishing touch to your silky legs and thighs. Johnson & Johnson produces the perenially favorite baby powder that most of us have used, or had used on us. And there was a good reason for Mom never dressing you before smoothing on plenty of sweet-smelling talcum powder all over your chubby little body. She knew that powder was beneficial in combating chafing in all those little folds and dimples that were so adorable when you were small. Well, you are much bigger now and certainly don't want any dimples, rolls or folds anywhere on your body. Even if you don't have any of that cute baby fat, chances are that your legs occasionally become chafed, particularly in the summertime. Chafing occurs when skin rubs against skin or skin against clothing. It can become painful if, for example, you wear a very tight pair of jeans in hot weather and perspire just a little. But a liberal application of talcum powder can certainly help to prevent that uncomfortable situation.

HAIR REMOVAL

Removing the hair on your legs and thighs is a personal decision. Some foreign cultures prize the look of a woman's legs with hair, whereas much of the "middle-class Western society" prefers to see women with smooth, hairless legs. In the 1970s, the early days of the recent feminist movement, leg shaving became a political issue much like bra burning. Many women refused to shave their legs because they believed this symbol of vanity to be dictated by men. Today, the political pendulum seems to have swung back to a more middle-of-the-road position, so the choice to shave or not to shave is no longer closely linked to one's politics. If you have decided that hair removal is for you, keep reading.

Depilatories

Those vile-smelling hair-removal concoctions of years past are quite thankfully gone forever. Taking their place are much milder, more pleasant-smelling creams that remove the hair efficiently and quickly. Depilatories work by dissolving the hair below the skin line. The chemicals in these lotions are powerful enough to break down the actual structure of the hair. All you do with a depilatory lotion is smooth it on the surface of the leg. It must remain on the skin for fifteen to twenty minutes; then wash off gently. The lotion and the hair will simply slide off, leaving the skin smooth and soft. It is a good idea to follow the instructions on the package; a patch test to determine your sensitivity to the alkaline chemicals in the depilatory lotion is always recommended. If you feel any itching, burning or see any redness during or after the patch test, do not use the depilatory; it is probably too harsh for your skin.

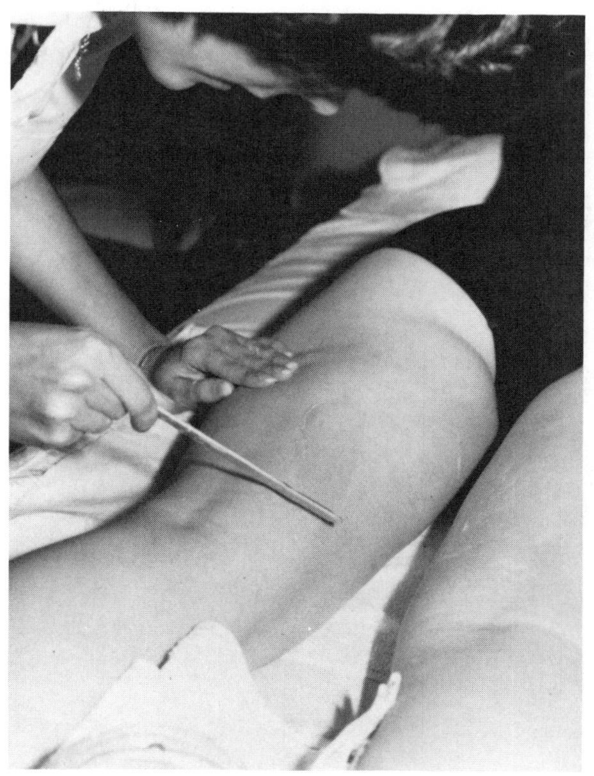

Liquid wax is applied to the skin.

Depilatories can be very messy and take some time to work, but they do leave the skin smooth and hair-free; because the hair is dissolved, it takes a week or longer to grow back. They are particularly effective at the sensitive "bikini line" where shaving is often too harsh.

Waxing

Although leg waxing is usually performed in salons that specialize in the procedure, it is possible to wax your legs at home, using one of

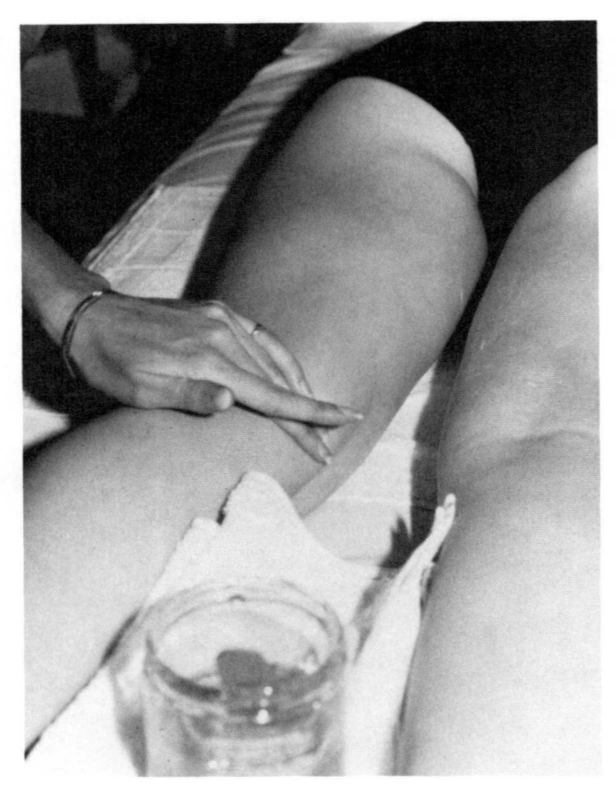

The wax is worked into the skin.

the packaged kits now available in pharmacies. The first time you do it, though, it's a good idea to have your legs professionally waxed.

Waxing is a process that actually pulls the hair out of its follicle. Warm, liquid wax is applied to the surface of the leg, and then strips of cloth are laid over the warm wax. As the wax sets, the hair is trapped in it, and when the cloth is pulled away, the wax and the hair are also pulled away from the leg. Waxing may sound like a primitive, painful experience, but it isn't nearly as bad as it sounds. Most skillful attendants work quickly, and the mildly stinging sensation is kept to a minimum.

Waxing, especially when performed professionally, can be expensive ($30 to 60 per session), somewhat painful, especially if you are particularly sensitive to the sensation, and it can be dangerous if you don't pay attention to what you're doing when you wax your legs at home. Remember that wax is extremely flammable and that it can burn your skin if it is applied when too hot. But it is a good alternative to a hair-removal solution, particularly if you find frequent shaving a real bother. Depending on

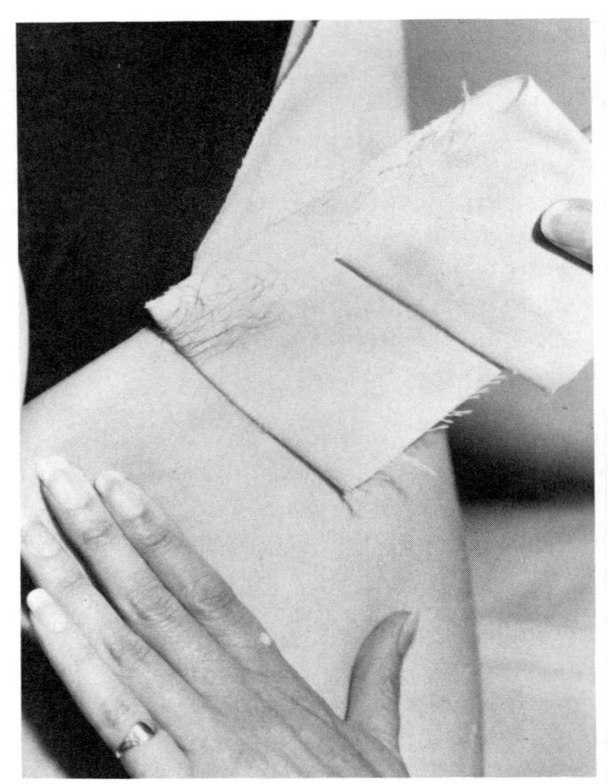

A cloth is applied to the still warm wax. Here the cloth is removed after the wax cools. Hair is pulled from its follicles.

your physical makeup, waxing can keep your legs smooth from ten to forty-five days.

Shaving

Leg shaving is probably more popular than all the other hair removal methods combined. Shaving is quick, fairly easy once you get the knack of it, and it's certainly inexpensive. If you decide to shave your legs, you have two choices, either to use an electric shaver or a razor. An electric shaver cuts the hair off above the skin line, so the legs don't stay smooth very long, which may pose a problem for you, especially if you're often short of time. Some women find shavers aesthetically unappealing because of the buzzing noise they make, but that's strictly a matter of taste.

Shaving with a razor is the most common shaving method, but it can be fraught with peril if you are hurried or haphazard about it. Every woman can remember the first time she shaved a layer of skin off her shin or ankle and watched in horror as the blood oozed to the surface and the bleeding wouldn't stop. Those nicks and cuts are rarely painful and certainly aren't dangerous, but they can leave scars. To

Pros and Cons of Hair-Removal Methods

Bleaching
Pros — quick; easy; makes soft, fine hair invisible.
Cons — temporary; chemicals can irritate the skin.

Shaving
Pros — quick; easy; does not damage follicle.
Cons — temporary; razors can cut skin.

Waxing
Pros — lasts from six to eight weeks; regrowth is slow.
Cons — frequent waxing can damage follicle and cause ingrown hairs; treatment is sometimes painful.

Depilatories
Pros — leaves legs smooth.
Cons — temporary; can be messy; chemicals break down structure of hair.

Tweezing
Pros — best temporary method for removing eyebrow hairs.
Cons — distorts follicle; stimulates regrowth; ingrown hairs possible.

Abrasion
Pros — simplest temporary method.
Cons — wears off skin.

Electrolysis
Pros — only permanent hair-removal method.
Cons — expensive; can be time-consuming; sometimes painful.

---

minimize the possibility of cutting or nicking your leg while shaving, take your time and use a layer of protective lather. Regular bath soaps work, but they may dry the skin; liquid shower soaps are better, but the best product is shaving cream. There's no rule that says those cans full of shaving lather are just for men, so give them a try. The creams lather on luxuriously and create a slick, wet surface that allows your razor to glide more easily against the skin. Shaving creams are available in all types of formulas and scents.

Another way to minimize your chances of cutting or scraping yourself is to always shave with a sharp blade. When you feel yours pulling or hesitating, it's time to change. Never share a razor or use one that's rusty or dull; if you do, you're asking for trouble.

Use particular care when you shave bumpy or bony areas like your knees, your ankles and your shins. And don't be in a hurry. If you decide to shave at the bikini line, use care not to shave too close; if you do, you will probably cause ingrown hairs and little bumps that can be very uncomfortable, especially in the summer heat. As mentioned previously, you might consider using a depilatory on this sensitive area.

SPECIAL TIPS FOR SUMMER

The long, lazy days of summer can be a real delight. They allow you extra daylight to enjoy all your favorite outdoor activities. But unless you take a few precautions, you could be setting yourself up for some real skin problems. Prolonged exposure to sunlight, of course, is very drying and damaging to your skin. It is of particular concern on your legs, because chances are you probably don't give them a second thought. When you're out bicycling, running or just picnicking, bare legs may receive a good amount of damaging sun rays. It is easy, though, to prevent major problems, just by paying attention and by using the proper sunscreen agent for your skin. Remember that as you perspire, your sunscreen will come off, so don't hesitate to apply more.

Areas that you should pay special attention to are your thighs, shins, knees and the backs of your knees. If you've ever been sunburned in any of those places, you know just how painful it can be.

When you're outdoors, if you notice your legs becoming bright red, blotchy or uncomfortable, cover them and head for the shade — fast. Summer's too short to have to spend time inside nursing a sunburn.

Remember, too, that the drying rays of the sun aren't the only weather element that will rob moisture from your skin. Wind, ocean air and the fact that you're probably exposing more length of leg to the hot air of summer will all help to damage your skin. So when you get back inside, be sure to apply plenty of moisturizing lotion to keep your skin soft and smooth.

WINTER WARNINGS

There's always a temptation in the wintertime to cut back on beauty routines you usually faithfully pursue during the rest of the year. After all, you might reason, "Nobody sees my legs under my tights, long pants or boots, so why should I bother?" But today's active woman can't afford to think that way — involvement in sports and taking care of your body doesn't go along with that kind of thinking. Besides, you're taking care of yourself as a personal commitment, aren't you? And you really don't want to look at your legs with dry skin, or if they're haphazardly groomed, just because no one else is looking. Resist the temptation to let go of your discipline. Remember PRIDE.

CLOTHING BEAUTY TIPS

There are all sorts of clever tricks that you can use to disguise the shape of your legs, if you feel that it's important enough to you. By far, the most common complaint that women have about their legs is that they are too heavy, too big, too stocky. So we're going to address primarily that problem. But we will also discuss how to dress for skinny legs.

Heavy Legs

Skirts. Your skirts shouldn't be too short or too tight. Strive for a soft look with some fullness to camouflage your figure. A lightly gathered dirndl skirt is probably your best bet. Your hemline is best at the upper end of your calf — that way you are able to take full advantage of your curves without revealing any bulges.

Shoes. A small heel always looks better than a flat on a heavy leg. The elevation of the heel gives a longer, leaner line. In general, the simpler the shoe, the better. Try classic pumps, loafers with a small heel (avoid very chunky heels, they'll only emphasize your chunky legs), boots and some sandals. Avoid shoes with ankle straps; they will cross your leg with a horizontal line and make them look bigger. Also avoid spiky heels; they'll emphasize your chunkiness.

When wearing casual outfits, such as shorts or tennis clothes, wear socklets instead of anklets, again to prevent that horizontal line from cutting your leg and making it look shorter and heavier.

Slacks and jeans. If you have heavy (saddlebag) thighs, avoid, at all costs, tight pants. If you wear tight pants, you'll only emphasize your figure problem. Keep those tight pants around, though; you're bound to lose those extra inches, and you'll soon be able to wear them comfortably again. In general, shop for clean, tailored lines with a minimum of fussy details. Avoid patch pockets, pleats, extra buckles and buttons, all of which will cause the eye to focus on those details — and right to your trouble spots. Instead, attempt to draw the eye upward by wearing attractive blouses with accessories like scarves, necklaces and fancy pins.

Jackets. It is very important when choosing a jacket that you get a good fit. Make sure that the jacket line crosses you at the most flattering point. That is, don't let it end just above or below your trouble spot — you'll only emphasize it. Instead, choose a well-tailored jacket that fits well and perhaps is nipped in a bit at the waist, extending just a little below the waist. You'll probably have to try on a number of jackets before you find the most flattering style, but do spend the time; the look will be worth it.

Stockings. Avoid fancy, patterned stockings if you're self-conscious about the size of your legs. Similarly, avoid light-colored tights and stockings. You should wear neutral or dark stockings. One of the most flattering looks is to wear a skirt, stockings and shoes in the same color. Burgundy, dark green, browns, navy blue and even black work well; do not use the same logic with colors like yellow, white or pink. You'll succeed only in making your legs look larger.

Shorts. Full, flared shorts are the most flattering style for heavy legs. The extra fabric softens and helps to hide what you don't want the world to see. Tight running shorts are best left to those with slim figures. If you're strong, solid and in shape, of course, feel free to wear running shorts that flatter your figure. You work hard for it — don't be afraid to show it off, if that's what you want to do in the appropriate situation.

Bathing suits. This may surprise you, but on heavy thighs, sometimes, a higher "French" cut looks best, since a longer-cut suit can make the leg appear shorter. As with most other clothing, you'll probably have to try on a number of different styles before you find the one that looks best on you. Look for the darker colors (they make you look slimmer), if you're at all self-conscious about your body.

Skinny Legs

Although the prevailing philosophy may be that you can never be too rich or too thin, there are probably many women agonizing just as much over their toothpick-thin legs as the women upset about their hefty ones. Again, although there's really not much you can do about changing your basic body structure, there are certain ways that you can fool the world and add visually to the bulk of your legs by dressing correctly.

Certainly, involvement in sports such as running, cycling and weight training can help you gain bulk and, in turn, add inches to your too-slim calves and thighs. But it takes a lot of work and careful attention to your program to add even an inch of muscle. Of course it's easier to add inches of fat to your body, especially to your legs and thighs, but that isn't a healthy course to gain weight. So before you start munching candy bars and sipping chocolate shakes to make your legs a bit fuller, consider the following eye-fooling tips.

Hosiery. Opaque stockings, patterned hose and outrageously bright knee socks and anklets were made for you! You can wear light colors, including whites and pastels, which will give the illusion of greater size and more bulk in your legs. Argyles and brightly patterned socks can add a fun touch to your casual outfits; don't be afraid to try them.

Pants. Thin legs look great in such fun fashions as knickers, short-cropped jeans and even bloomer-type pants. Wide, full, drawstring pants help to cover your thin legs, and also give the illusion of greater size.

In general, you can get away with wearing those fashions that many women would love to — and there are plenty of very fun, casual fashions available these days that will flatter your thinner figure. If you like the way they look and feel on you, very skinny, French-cut jeans might just be your choice; they'll certainly make you feel very continental, and you'll probably be the envy of your larger friends.

Skirts. The rule with skirts is to avoid calling too much attention to your legs if you're at all self-conscious about them. But if you like them thin, just the way they are, then let them show! Today's outrageous fashions: New Wave mini-skirts, short peasant skirts and long sweatshirts that are really short dresses. They are attractive on the thin-legged figure. Try them teamed with a pair of patterned socks and flat shoes for the most up-to-date look you can get.

Shoes. When you purchase shoes consider proportion. If your legs are spindly, you don't want to pick clunky shoes that make your legs appear even thinner. Instead, pick a more modified shoe with cleaner lines. You can wear very thin, almost spiked heels, if they are comfortable and attractive to you. And shoes without heels are very flattering to a thinner leg; the lack of a heel brings the leg down and alludes to bigger size. You probably should avoid platform sandals, both for aesthetic reasons and because they only accentuate the thinness. The same applies to clogs.

Shorts. Short shorts, long shorts, culottes; for you almost anything goes. Unless you are very self-conscious about your legs being extremely thin, you can wear skimpy running shorts in a variety of colors. Pastel colors add more illusion of weight, as, of course, whites also do. Very baggy shorts will tend to accentuate your thinness, so your choices should be more form-fitting (not tight) and of clingy rather than stiff fabrics.

Remember, you can't change your basic anatomy, so learn to live with it and enjoy your body for what it is; as the old Joe South song says, "Won't somebody please take the woman with the skinny legs?"

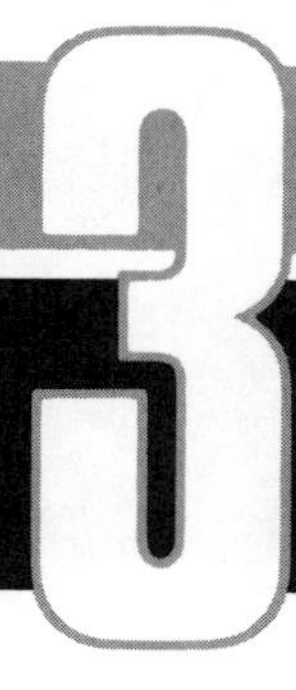

BASICS OF ANATOMY

Living in the modern world, clothed and muffled, forced to convey our sense of our bodies in terms of remote-symbols like walking sticks and umbrellas and handbags, it is easy to lose sight of the immediacy of the human body plan.

— Margaret Mead

There are certain facts about human anatomy and physiology that help us to understand how to maximize our physical potential. Man (used generically) evolved as a bipedal (two-legged stride) creature at least four million years ago when *Australopithecus,* a forerunner to modern man, first strode the earth on two legs. Man is the only primate to use bipedal locomotion as his primary means of movement. (There are those cynics who would argue that the automobile has really replaced bipedalism.) In any case, the ability to walk around on two legs was the result of the survival of those who were fittest — a la Charles Darwin and the theory of natural selection. Therefore, we who have survived have made that adaptation which, for our species, has been the most successful.

One of the adaptations that has taken place has been in the length, size and structure of the leg — which must be long in proportion to the rest of the body to allow one to both balance and to stride. This information may help you to understand why we're built the way we are and why it helps so much to keep your body in shape — the shape in which it was intended to be in order to maintain optimum strength, flexibility and efficiency.

THE FOUNDATION — BONES

Your basic body structure is largely determined by your body's framework, your skeletal network of 206 bones. The muscles, ligaments, tendons, organs and fat are all draped around, between and among the bones. Your potential size and shape is mostly determined by your bone structure — and that was genetically ordained at the moment of conception. Therefore, there's really nothing you can do about being 5 feet 8 inches if you are 5 feet 2 inches. What you can control, to a certain extent, is the way that those 5 feet 2 inches take shape; how much fat how much muscle, and, ultimately, the size, strength and bulk of those muscles. But your bone structure is set — you can recognize that fact and move on, or you can spend much of your time wishing for the impossible.

Of the 206 bones in your body, surprisingly few make up the structure of the leg. The bones of the leg, because they must support the weight of the entire body, are very strong and heavy. The femur (the largest bone in your body) extends from the pelvis to the knee; the somewhat smaller fibula and tibia extend from

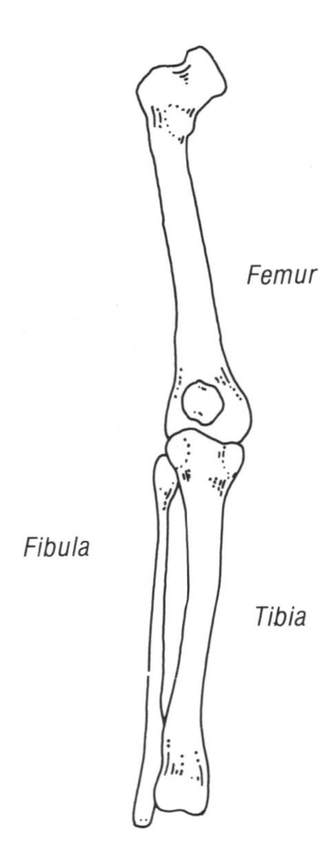

Bones of the leg.

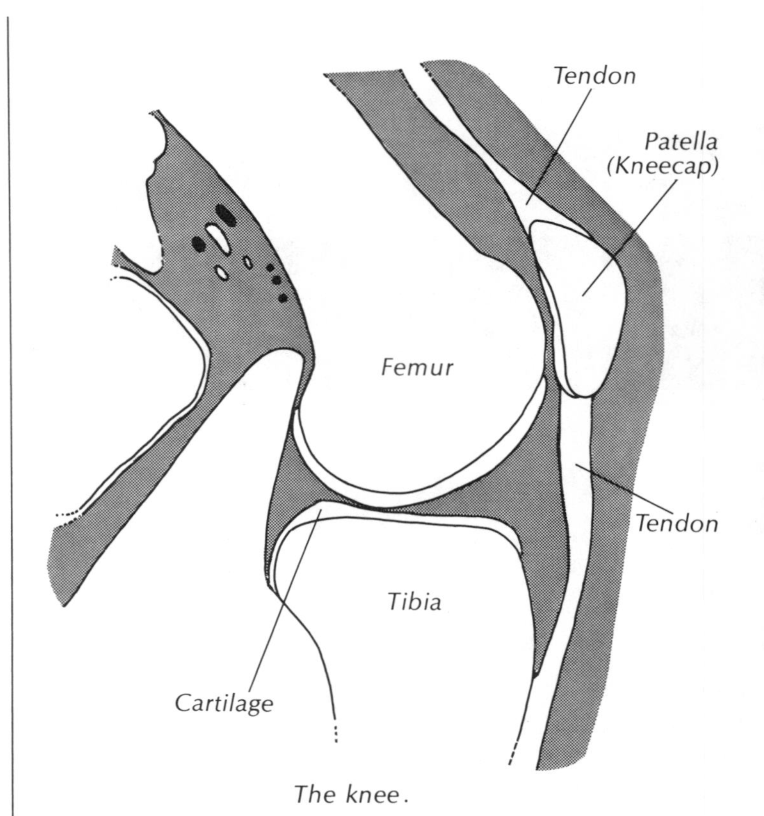

The knee.

the knee to the ankle, and the patella (kneebone) covers the joint where the three major bones join.

As you probably remember from childhood, Mom always made you drink your milk and finish your meal. Well, she was right. Milk is a good source of calcium, which gives bones their strength and rigidity. And vitamins and other minerals in food supply the blood vessel networks that nourish the bone and keep them oxygenated.

THE HINGES — JOINTS

Your body's framework is held together by a series of ingeniously designed joints. We require smooth-working joints, otherwise we would all be walking around like stiff-legged Frankensteins! Since that wasn't the plan for man, we've been lucky enough to have developed many types of joints, each appropriate to the function for which it was designed. Think about the way that your hip bone connects to your pelvis bone, and then think about how your arm bones are connected at the elbows. Quite specific differences, aren't there? There are seven different types of joints in your body: hinge (elbow), ball and socket (hip and shoulder), pivot (head and neck), saddle (ankle), condylar (knee), ellipsoid (wrist) and plane (between the toes).

Knee

The knee is one of the most abused areas of the entire body. We all know an athlete who has had or is contemplating knee surgery, and the ranks of tennis players, runners and basketball stars are replete with athletes bearing knee scars. Why so many knee injuries? First, the knee is a complex and delicate joint comprised of tendons, ligaments and cartilage. Second, knees are subjected to more stresses than any joint in the body. Consider the stop-and-go action of basketball, or the pounding from running on pavement. Third, this is a weight-bearing joint.

Many knee injuries occur when the knee is extended, then accidentally twisted. That's because the joint has less range of motion than the ankle or wrist joints, for example. Knee injuries can be painful and are often discouraging, because they are usually slow to heal. And to heal, they require a reduction in activity. However, a sport like swimming is good to pursue during the healing stage. You can maintain aerobic fitness without stressing the bad knee.

As with so many problems, preventive measures go a long way. Be sure to warm up before starting your exercise routine. Stretch and do some jogging before you exercise intensely. The importance of strengthening your quadriceps can't be underemphasized. Weight training will strengthen and improve the flexibility of the quadriceps, which literally keep your knee joint together. The stronger the quadriceps, the less weight bearing your knee joint must accept.

What should you do if you do have knee pains or problems? If your pain is chronic, consult a physician, preferably one with an interest in sportsmedicine. Don't aggravate your condition by refusing to deal with it; learn from your doctor about how much and what types of exercise are best for you. Although many athletes bear scars from knee surgery, it isn't always necessary to repair a torn ligament, a stretched tendon or damaged cartilage; strides are being made with a surgical procedure that enables the physician to make only minimal incisions, through the use of fiber optics. If your doctor recommends any type of surgical procedure, it's wise to get a second opinion before making a commitment.

Minor knee problems can be dealt with by following the RICE method of treatment (see Chapter 5). The knee usually needs rest after an injury. Overuse injuries, especially, call for backing off on your training.

THE MOVING FORCE — MUSCLES

C'mon, make a muscle! How many times have you heard that challenge since you were a child? Muscles are visible evidence of the way we treat our bodies, of how much attention we pay to exercise and diet. Muscles are one of the very first body parts to respond to the right (or wrong) kind of treatment. Have you ever had a broken bone and had to wear a cast for eight weeks? If so, you'll remember how atrophied and withered the limb looked when the cast was removed. The reason for the atrophy was lack of use. That's a very graphic, vivid example, and the truth is that if you don't keep physically active, your muscles will waste away.

Perhaps a more universal analogy is to ask you to remember the last time that you had a bout with the flu. Remember how weak and tired you felt, the first day back to your regular routine? Some of that dragged-out-feeling was caused by the nature of the illness, but much of it was the loss of muscle tone after a week or so of just lying around. No, muscles do not automatically "turn to fat," but they do become flabby and weakened, losing their previous strength after only a few days of not being used. That's why exercise programs stress the importance of doing something four or five days a week, rather than saving yourself and going for it only on weekends.

Now that you know the importance of regular use, you might like to know just what it is that muscles do and what their structure is all about. Basically, muscles are bundles of fibers attached to each other in four different ways: spiral (trapezius in the back), triangular (pectoralis in the chest), strap-like (sartorius in the leg) and multipennate (deltoids in the arm). As with the hinge structures found in the joints, muscle structures are specifically designed to maximize performance and the function for which they were created. An example is the difference between the large and powerful gluteus maximus (more maximus in some than in others!) designed to move the entire leg, and the delicate muscles in the face, such as the risorius, that move the mouth.

Muscles move by contraction. The contractions in certain muscles can be up to one-third the length of the muscle. Muscles, while they are arranged singularly, most often function in groups that work in opposition to each other — that is, when one muscle (or muscle group) contracts, the other (opposing) group expands. This principle of muscle movement is responsible for your ability to bend and flex your limbs. An example of muscles in your legs that work in opposition to each other is the combination of gastrocnemius (the back of the calf)

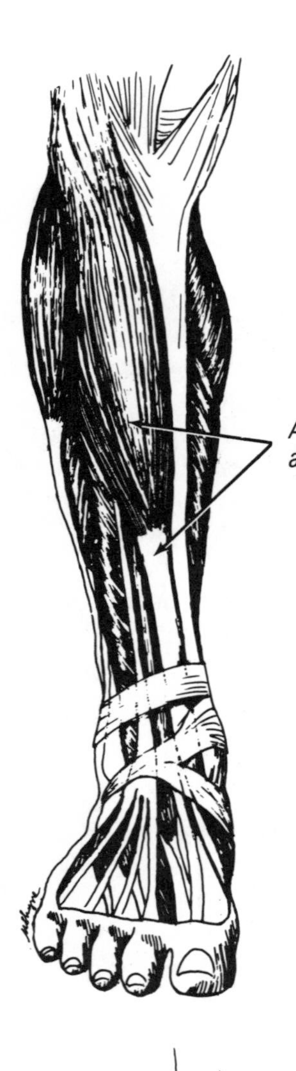

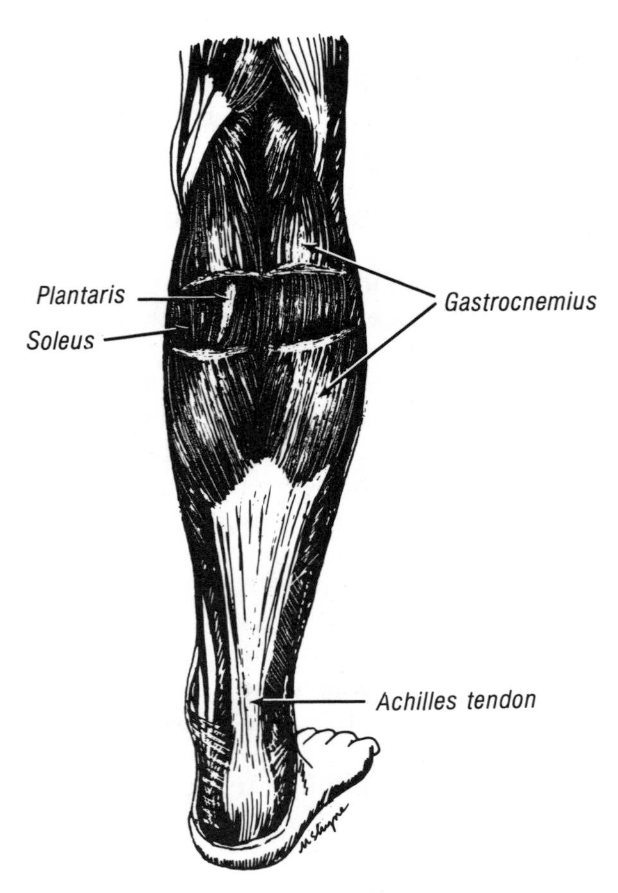

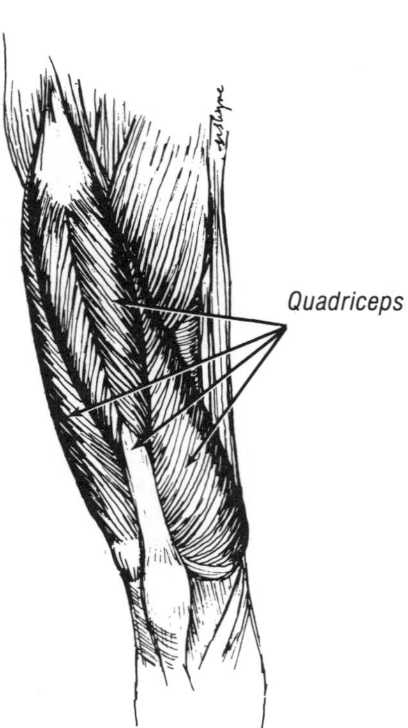

Front leg muscles.

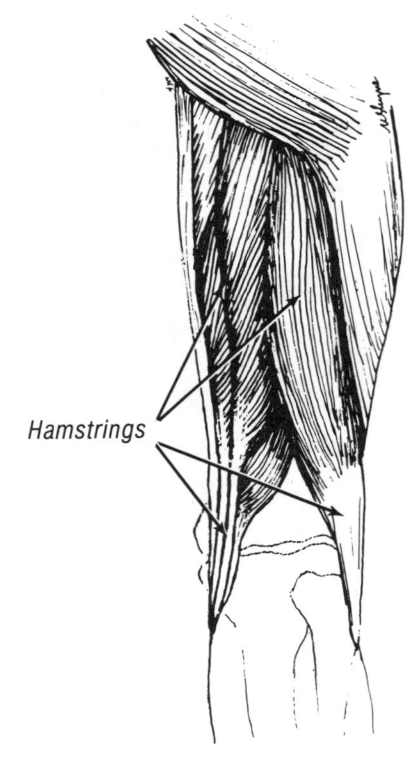

Back leg muscles.

and the tibialis anterior (the muscle in the front of the lower leg). If you work the calf muscle and don't also work the tibialis, you can create a muscle imbalance, where one set is much stronger than the other complementary set of muscles. This condition can be painful, and in this particular situation results in the condition known as shinsplints. The common remedy for muscle imbalances is to build up the less-conditioned set of muscles.

Lucky for you, muscles are easy to build and condition — you have all seen the famous Charles Atlas ads where he claimed to have once been a ninety-seven-pound weakling. Undertaking a major muscle-building program gave him a remarkably strong and well-defined body. Of course, you probably have no desire to add the type of muscle development to your frame that Charles Atlas did, but then probably no one has ever kicked sand in your face, either. In fact, you simply cannot build Charles Atlas muscles, because of your female hormones. More about muscle building later.

Muscles exhibit certain characteristics of fitness, which indicate their tone and ability to respond to given situations. Those characteristics include:

Flexibility — amount of suppleness and ability to stretch.

Strength — the ability of a muscle to exert tension against resistance.

Speed — the ability to quickly contract through the range of motion, recover and repeat the motion.

Endurance — the ability of a muscle to repeat specific motions.

It is possible to increase each characteristic of muscle tone through exercise; however, there are certain limits based upon one's frame size, genetic inheritance and certain environmental factors, such as the amount of stress and the type of diet you pursue in your daily activity.

Flexibility can be increased by doing a number of stretching exercises, by practicing yoga and, basically, by paying attention to your movement. Increase the amount of stretching you do very gradually and always remember, do not bounce! Bouncing when you stretch can injure your muscles.

Strength can be improved by the repetition of a given exercise. That's why, for instance, if you spend your entire summer riding your bicycle instead of driving your car, you'll discover that your legs are very strong by Labor Day. You've repeated the same movement time and time again, so your muscles have become more efficient at repeating that movement. To increase strength, you must increase the resistance on your muscles for a given activity. Strength is best gained in weight lifting by lifting a heavy weight (for your level of ability) a few times. So do a few sets of lifts using a heavy weight.

Contrary to popular belief, you can increase your speed, although it's true that some people are born to be fast and others are born to be slow. That's because we are endowed with a certain ratio of muscles — fast twitch and slow twitch. Fast-twitch muscles predominate in those who are good sprinters; endurance athletes have a preponderance of slow-twitch muscles. You cannot change the slow-twitch/fast-twitch ratio. But you can increase your speed in any sport such as running, swimming or cycling by working on your speed by training hard and fast. This will allow you to reach your potential.

Endurance, or the ability of the muscle to repeat a movement over and over for an extended period of time, is another muscle characteristic that can be improved through practice. The idea is to work up to it gradually. If you lift weights, you should do a large number of repetitions using a light weight (for your ability). The important factor with building endurance is volume, or number of repetitions, no matter what your sport.

Each of the characteristics of muscle fitness is easy to work on — once you're determined to develop your muscle tone, to a point where you can feel the muscle, but not in a painful way. If you feel a painful twinge when attempting a specific stretch or movement, stop immediately and back off. Pain is an indication that you're doing too much, too soon. No pain, no gain may be a modern maxim, but it's one that you shouldn't listen to unless you're really a masochist at heart.

The same goes for speedwork, strength training and building endurance. Your body will tell you when you've had enough, and it's important to recognize the fundamental difference between real pain and just discomfort.

No two pain thresholds are alike in people. Generally, the more experience you have with exercise, the greater your pain threshold. It's important that you learn, based on your body's responses, what will cause pain, what will cause discomfort and what you just resist doing because you're lazy, too tired or just not feeling like performing on a given day. Mostly, this comes from experience. There are no formulas, no machines that can tell you when to stop for your own good. What's important, though, is that you follow your own feelings, and not try to copy someone else's workout schedule. Her pain threshold may be greater than yours. Comparing yourself to someone else is asking for trouble.

If you wake up one morning with sore muscles, or a tendon or joint that just doesn't feel right, think about the possible causes. Remember what you did to make yourself sore. Did you overdo it? Usually soreness is the result of extending the muscle beyond its trained level. When you begin an exercise program some soreness is to be expected. But with time, soreness will go away and only come back in unusual situations. You might use a muscle improperly, for example. Or you might take up another type of exercise that stresses muscles not normally used (trained) in your other activity.

SKIN

Your skin is an organ, the largest one in your body. It makes up nearly 7 percent of your body weight and receives a rich blood supply from the cardiovascular system. The skin both protects and senses, enabling you to detect pain, heat and cold, pressure and touch. Additionally, the skin functions as an elimination organ, responsible for producing perspiration, which cools the body when it is overheated.

Think about just how sensitive your skin is — how it can readily detect the difference between a swatch of burlap and a swatch of silk; the difference between a hot iron and a piece of ice. Your skin is loaded with thousands of nerve receptors, which allow you to make those differentiations instantly, but sometimes we don't receive warnings from our body's defense mechanisms until it is too late. Remember the last time that you had a bad sunburn, a case of chapped or windburned skin? Skin problems can usually be prevented by just being prepared for the daily situations that might damage it. Overexposure to sunlight, wind, cold air and even to harsh chemicals (like chlorinated water) can dry the skin, resulting in chapping and rough and scaly patches.

Proper skin care, then, should be your priority, both for your general health and for your beauty. Understanding the basics about skin structure will help to improve your ability to care for it.

Your skin is comprised of a number of layers; the epidermis alone is made of five layers of cells, which are specifically designed to protect you from the elements. The first line of defense in keeping your skin healthy, soft and supple is to keep it moisturized. You can do that in two ways: by ingesting enough water to keep it hydrated (full of water), and by applying lotions and creams to keep the moisture in the skin, rather than allowing it to evaporate through exposure to the elements. Just be sure to include plenty of water in your diet — either by drinking water, juices and herbal teas or by eating plenty of healthy, fresh vegetables and fruits. Those moisture-rich foods will also nourish your body by providing plenty of vitamins, minerals and fiber, which will help your skin to glow.

The reason your skin needs moisture is to help it to function properly. The body, as you probably already know, is composed of mostly water. Water lubricates the delicate tissues, allows for elimination of waste products and provides the necessary medium for essential minerals, and other nutrients to be carried throughout the body. You've heard of people surviving in the desert without food for days, but not without water — it clearly is our most precious resource.

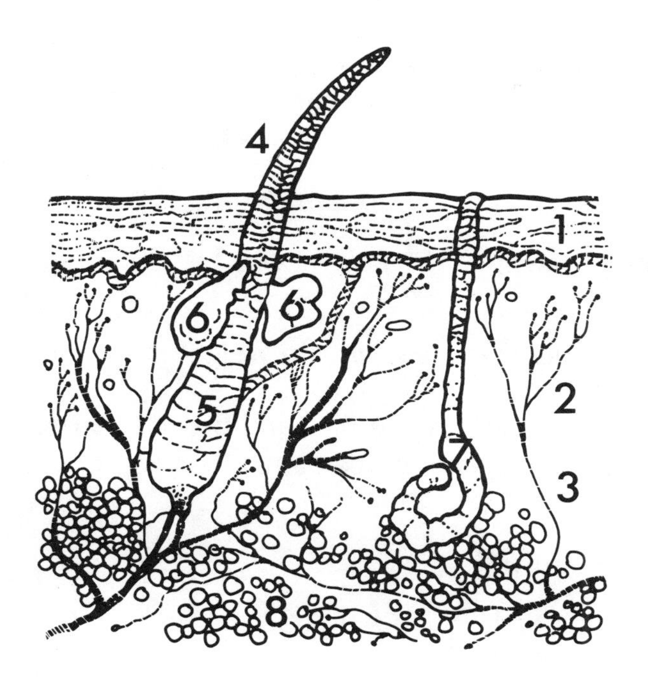

1. Epidermis
2. Dermis
3. Hypodermis
4. Hair shaft
5. Hair follicle
6. Sebaceous (oil) gland
7. Sudoriferous (sweat) gland
8. Blood vessels

Despite the claims of many product ads, special creams and lotions cannot put moisture back into your skin, but they can help to seal in the moisture that you already have. That's why you'll get the best results if you apply a moisturizer when your skin is still a bit damp from your daily shower or bath.

Daily bathing, of course, is a must for good skin care. Washing the skin removes surface dirt and bacteria, washes away the dead surface cells on your skin that can give it a dull appearance and, while it doesn't actually allow the skin to "breathe," it is refreshing.

BODY TYPES

As we've mentioned, it's important to realize your body's potential, and while setting reasonable goals, understand that there are some limitations over which you have no control. One of the easy ways that we can categorize the size and shape of your ideal body is called "somatyping." Basically, there are three basic body types:

1. Endomorph
2. Mesomorph
3. Ectomorph

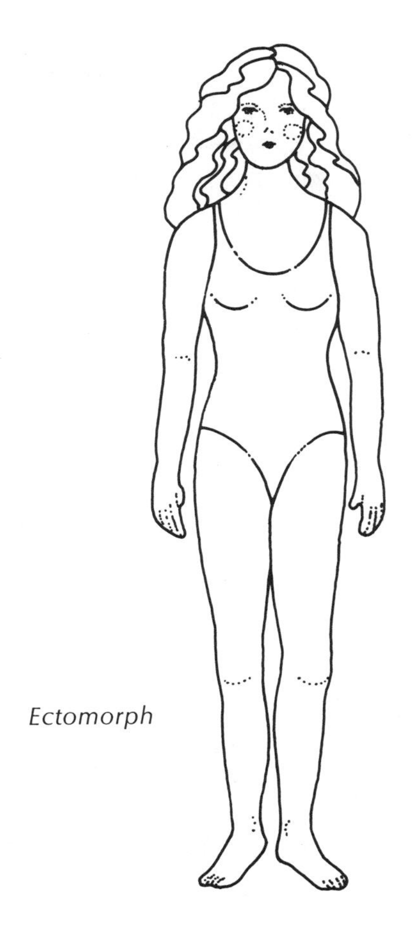
Ectomorph

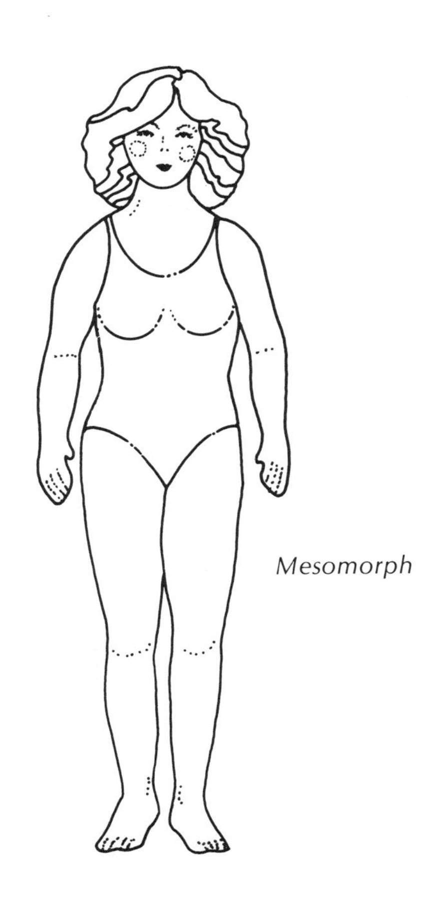
Mesomorph

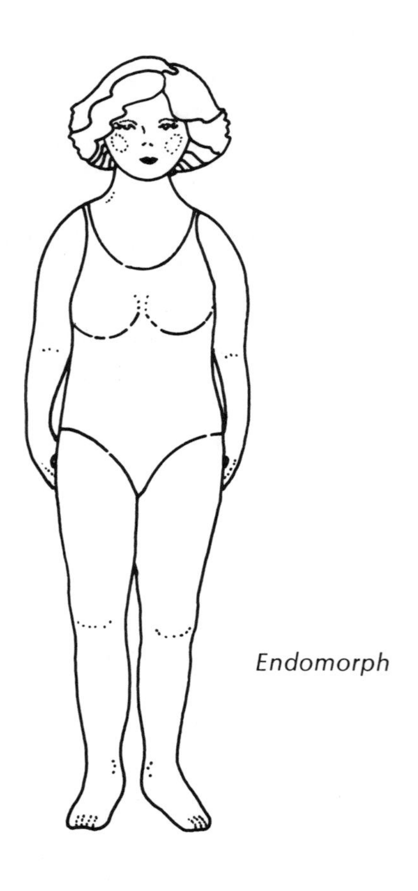

Endomorph

Each of these three body types has clear-cut characteristics that are fairly obvious when a body is in good shape. Of course, it's possible for a person who is overweight or underweight or out of shape to obscure her basic body type.

Endomorph

— rounded body
— tendency to readily gain weight in the form of fat
— large bones, wide hips and broad shoulders
— the higher the percentage of fat, the poorer the athletic performance

Mesomorph

— muscular body
— stocky build
— little fat

Ectomorph

— linear build (often "tall and stringy")
— prominent bones
— fragile appearance
— little fat

4 FOOD, FABULOUS FOOD

Eat to live, but do not live to eat.
— *Ben Franklin*

In 1982, an article in *California* magazine, by Elizabeth Kaye, stated brilliantly, "There may be something better than eating. But what?" Indeed, many American women (and men) have an emotional, love/hate relationship with food. We get crazy when we're hungry. We eat at every social occasion; we eat when we're bored, lonely, scared or depressed. We stuff ourselves on holidays, at the movies; we do it to please our mothers. But we seldom pause to think about what it is that we're putting into our bodies.

Remember the gallows-type humor of Valerie Harper when, as the character Rhoda Morgenstern, she would laughingly take a doughnut, cake or other sweet and say, "I don't know why I'm eating this. I may just as easily apply it directly to my hips." Valerie Harper has reduced the size of her hips now, presumably out of an awareness that there was, indeed, a relationship between what goes into one's mouth and what appears on one's hips. Or thighs.

Because of our genetic makeup and our biological inheritance, we seem to be walking targets for excess flesh accumulating on our hips, thighs and buttocks. Many women have a real problem with fat settling on the thighs, just below the buttocks — the "saddlebag thighs."

What is it that causes that accumulation of fat? You pay attention to your diet and you try to get enough exercise; what is it that's going wrong? The formula is a simple mathematical equation. And for those of you who cringe at the thought of math, this equation is easier than you may think. First, a pound of fat equals 3500 calories. Therefore, to gain one pound of fat, you must take in 3500 calories more than you burn. Conversely, if you are to lose one pound of fat, you must take in 3500 calories fewer than you did previously. Or, in terms of exercise, you can gain one pound of fat by reducing your activity level by 3500 calories, or you can lose one pound of fat by increasing your activity level by 3500 calories.

Yes, but what does that mean in terms of my daily diet/exercise routine you may ask? Simple. Your daily caloric needs for basic body functions (depending on your height and weight) are between 1800 and 2000 per day. If you participate in no exercise that day and eat right at 1800 to 2000 calories, your body will not accumulate any extra calories — hence you will experience no change in your weight.

If, however, you take in 2500 calories, then your body will have taken in at least 500 calories more than it needed that day. If you do no extra exercise to account for that extra calorie intake, the excess will be stored as, you guessed it, fat. If you accumulate 3500 calories, that caloric excess will appear on the scales (and on your body) as one extra pound.

Conversely, if you burn more calories than you take in, you will lose a corresponding amount of excess calories (known as fat). Go for an extra-long run (burning calories at the rate of one hundred per mile) and you'll burn more calories than you usually do. Consider, also, that even after you've finished your run you continue to burn calories (for several hours) at an elevated rate, which is increasing your basal metabolism. It's really pretty easy to manage your weight, once you get the knack of figuring out your daily caloric needs and balancing them with your caloric expenditures.

Weight (Pounds)	**Maintenance Calorie Intake** (Low to Moderate Activity)
87-100	1400
101-114	1600
115-126	1800
127-139	2000
140-153	2200
154-166	2400
167-179	2600
180-193	2800

Source: **The California Diet and Exercise Program.** Anderson World Books, Inc., 1983, by Dr. Peter Wood. Reprinted with permission.

A prominent magazine publisher was known to keep track of his daily calorie intake, making sure to run at least eight miles per day so that he could consume a banana split daily; he was at his ideal weight and dearly loved the high-calorie treat, so in order to enjoy food without gaining weight, he earned his banana split each day. This is, however, not recommended. In addition to watching your calories, you must watch the nutritional content of your food. His high-fat, high-sugar habit didn't make him fat, but it wasn't good for him, either.

Contrary to any emotional feelings you may have about food, food is simply fuel. Food is burned for energy, and there are certain types of food that are more efficient sources of fuel than others. The government-approved basic four food groups have been recommended for decades. You should balance your diet with the proper number of daily helpings from the basic four food groups.

Portion sizes can tell a lot; did you know, for instance, that one-half bagel serves as one carbohydrate serving? Or how about two tablespoons of raisins? Both examples are known as "calorie-dense" foods; that is, they pack a lot of calories for their size. It's important to know both the nutritional value and the caloric content of your food. That way, you'll find out that a high-fat, high-salt splurge at your local hamburger stand should be done only rarely.

Foods high in carbohydrates have been unjustly maligned as high-calorie foods. For the athletic or active woman, foods high in carbohydrates provide good, plentiful sources of energy. In fact, one of the most disdained of all vegetables, the lowly potato, is a very healthy food, rich in vitamin C and many minerals. It's only when you smother it in butter, sour cream or heaps of Cheddar cheese that it becomes a fattening food. In fact, according to nutritionists, an ideal, high-nutrient meal is a baked potato topped with a scoop of low-fat cottage cheese.

The subject of nutrition belongs in any exercise book. Proper nutrition is what keeps you going strong; it helps determine whether you'll win or lose and how you'll feel while you play the game. Spend some time reading and learning about good nutrition; you're sure to experience some revelations about your own food habits. And if eating food is a source of emotional stress for you, as in binge eating, anorexia nervosa or eating to please others, don't suffer through your problem in silence. Many people have the same problems; get some help from a professional group. Food can be an addiction worse than alcohol or drugs because it's a substance you can't live without. You're faced with it every day. Learning how to deal with it can be a blessing.

FOUR BASIC FOOD GROUPS

For optimum nutrition, you should choose the appropriate portions of your daily food intake from the four basic food groups. Calories count, but so does nutrition, so make sure that you get the most from your diet by making well-informed food choices every time you sit down to a meal.

Milk Group. This group provides you with calcium, B vitamins and riboflavin, in addition to vitamin A and protein. Depending on your choices, the milk group can allow you to cut a great deal of fat from your diet. Pay attention to labels and concentrate on purchasing low-fat or nonfat milk, cheeses and yogurt. You'll notice that the fat content percentages in your milk-group foods have no effect on the nutritional content. So be good to your heart, your arteries and your waistline by selecting low-fat (and in the case of yogurts) low-sugar foods. Ice cream, cottage cheese and chocolate milk are other choices. Adults should get two or more servings daily.

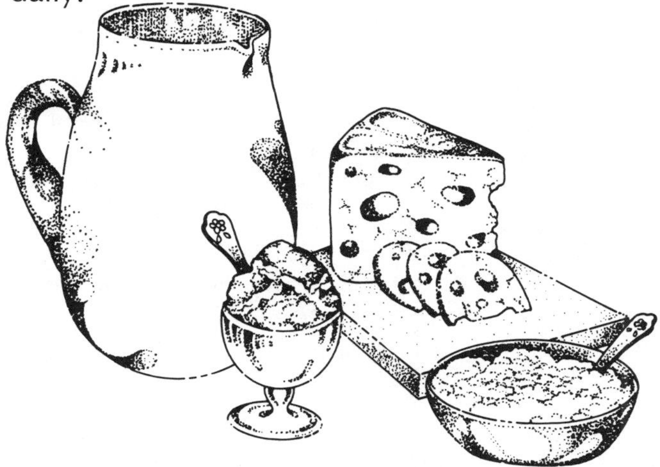

Meat Group. You need not be a carnivore to make food choices from the so-called "meat group." Basically, this group supplies you with your daily supply of protein, the basic building blocks for tissue development. You can get all the protein you need by making sensible combinations of vegetables and legumes, including beans, peanuts (and peanut butter), eggs, soybeans and tofu. Cheese is a good source of protein, as well. If you prefer to eat meat, your wisest choices are poultry (without the skin) and fish, which are high in protein but low in fat and cholesterol. Most red meat is difficult to digest and high in fat. You should have at least two servings from this group each day.

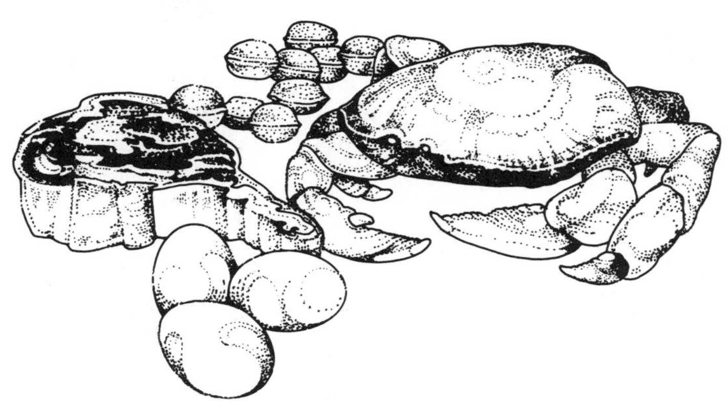

Vegetables and Fruits. Fruits and vegetables are excellent sources of vitamins, particularly A and C. They also provide you with fiber and low-calorie, eye-pleasing taste treats. In general, the deeper the color of the food, the more nutrient-packed it will be. Choose dark-green lettuce, deep-purple plums and vibrantly orange carrots, for example. One of the great things about fruits and vegetables is that they are filling and yet low in calories. Plan for four servings daily.

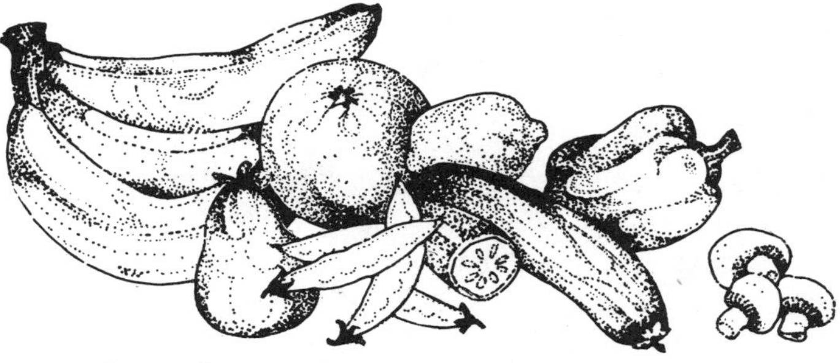

Breads and Cereals. Whole grain cereals are your best source of B vitamins and many minerals. Concentrate on cooking with and purchasing whole grain breads, cereals, muffins and grains like oats, rice and bulgur wheat. With a little experimentation, you'll learn to appreciate the nutty flavor of whole grains. They are versatile, chewy and very delicious, in addition to being packed with important nutrients. They are a superior form of complex carbohydrates, important for the athlete who is training. Eat four or more servings daily.

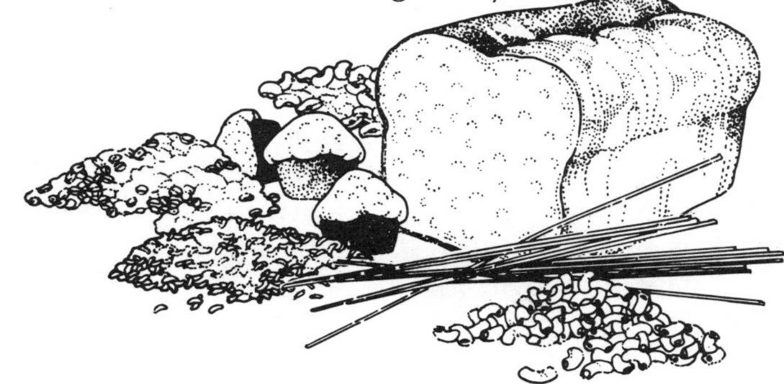

How Much Should You Weigh?

Height	Low Pounds	Weight Average Pounds	High Pounds
5′	100	109	118
5′ 1″	104	112	121
5′ 2″	107	115	125
5′ 3″	110	118	128
5′ 4″	113	122	132
5′ 5″	116	125	135
5′ 6″	120	129	139
5′ 7″	123	132	142
5′ 8″	126	136	146
5′ 9″	130	140	151
5′ 10″	133	144	156
5′ 11″	137	148	161
6′	141	152	166

FOOD AS MUSCLE FUEL

To understand the need for proper nutrition in the daily diet, it's important that you know the basics about metabolism — the way your body burns energy. Basically, muscles run on glycogen, which is a chemical derivative of digested and stored carbohydrates. Throw away all those notions you may have about starches (carbohydrates) being too fattening to eat. Complex carbohydrates are the richest source of energy for your muscles. Whole grain breads, cereals, pastas, potatoes, rice and fruit are all good sources of complex carbohydrates. Since your muscles can't store a supply of glycogen that will get you through the entire day, it's important to make sure that your daily intake of carbohydrates is constant so that it is resupplied. If you know that you're going to be extremely active, sometimes it's a good idea to eat an extra piece of fruit or bread to give you an extra supply of energy. You've probably heard about competitive athletes who practice carbohydrate loading. It's a deliberate attempt to saturate the body with carbohydrates for a week before a competitive event. Come race day, then, the muscles will take that much longer to burn off their supply of readily available supply of glycogen in the form of carbohydrates. After that, the body burns fat, which is not as easy on the body because the conversion process of fat to energy is inefficient.

As far as metabolism goes, remember that the old idea of a high-protein, low-carbohydrate diet is not right for an active woman. High-protein diets tend to be difficult to digest. They dehydrate the body because they utilize so much water in the digestion process, and they just don't provide you with enough quick energy. So forget the idea that eating steak and foregoing the baked potato is a good practice for an athletic person. In fact, just the opposite is true. Eat the baked potato, but not a plateful of meat. Most red meat has too much fat.

To have a smooth-running metabolic process, eat plenty of complex carbohydrates, minimize your fat intake and drink plenty of water to aid your muscles' efficiency in utilizing the stores of glycogen. Water is essential for the proper functioning of chemical reactions in metabolism. Water both supplies the needed oxygen and carries away the waste products created in metabolism. Keep your body hydrated at all times and remember to drink water *before* you're thirsty when you're involved in sports.

The food you eat can be compared to the type of fuel you put into your car's gas tank. If you have a Porsche, you certainly don't want to put watered-down gasoline into it — you want to give it the best high-performance fuel you can get. The same goes for your body — you don't want to junk it up by putting lots of fat into it, to clog up your fuel lines (arteries and veins); eat high-carbohydrate foods, which are like premium gas to a car.

How to Avoid a Binge

There are times when you will not eat properly, when you will bow to temptation and have that banana split, indulge in two more pieces of pizza than you really want (or need) or celebrate a birthday with just one more piece of cake. Don't fret. An occasional "treat" won't hurt you, and it will go a long way in allowing you to feel that you are in control of your eating habits. But you may be one of those people who equates food with emotional factors in her life and learns that food is a friend who will always be there during the long, lonely hours you may spend alone. If that is your situation, it's important that you recognize your behavior and learn alternative ways to fill your time. Here are some suggestions:

1. Take a class. Any class. In fact, take something that is completely outside of your everyday world. Don't know a thing about rocks? Take a geology class. Spend all your time doing very physical activities? Take a poetry class. The objective here is to grow — to extend your horizons and widen your vision.

2. Rearrange your furniture. Hang a photo of a special friend, clean out your dresser drawers. Throw yourself into a task that needs to be done, but for which you can find every excuse in the world not to do. Do it!

3. Call a friend and plan an activity. Not lunch. Plan to get together to go shopping, play a set of tennis or backgammon, or just to talk for a while. You'll find that when you are with company, you'll focus your thoughts on a person rather than food.

4. Keep your food diary up-to-date and realize that if you stuff yourself, you'll have to write it down. Do you really want to read about eating a package of Oreos or a quart of Haagen-Dazs?

5. Put on a leotard and tights and work out for a while. Invest in a tape or record of your favorite aerobic superstar and then do it! Learn the routine so well that the music is your cue; you don't even need to think about what comes next.

6. Go outside and play. No matter what the weather, a walk in the fresh air will help you take your mind off eating and put it back on living. Notice the houses as you pass by them: How would you paint them/change them/landscape them if one of them were yours? Let your mind wander and enjoy this beautiful world we live in.

7. Drink a glass of mineral water. Buy yourself a fancy crystal goblet that you use when you're feeling especially low. Fill it with ice cubes and mineral water, topped off by a squeeze of lime or a sprig of mint. How refreshing, filling and non-caloric!

8. Get your favorite magazine, a fluffy towel and some bubble bath and take a long, luxurious soak in the tub.

9. Write a letter to a friend who you've been meaning to write to but just can't find the time — now you have the time.

10. Pull out the atlas and find an exotic place where you would like to vacation. Plan the entire trip, from making reservations to packing your bags.

There are thousands of other ways that you can keep yourself from participating in compulsive behavior that you don't want to be part of your life. You can be in control of whatever you want in your life — just make it clear what you want and go after it!

EASY SUBSTITUTIONS YOU CAN MAKE

The following are suggestions for paring calories from your diet.

• Substitute yogurt for sour cream in virtually any recipe. For additional benefit, use nonfat yogurt.

• Eat a baked apple instead of a piece of apple pie.

• Eat fruit rather than drinking the juice — fruit has more bulk and takes longer to digest.

• Eat baked potatoes rather than french fries.

• Use thin salad dressings, enabling you to use much less than the creamy types. Or, better yet, use just a squeeze of lemon, tomato juice or a dressing without an oil base.

• Choose dense, whole grain breads and rolls rather than airy, white breads. Whole grains are chewier, and not nutritionally depleted.

• If you drink whole milk, switch to low-fat. If you drink low-fat, switch to nonfat.

• If you like tuna fish, switch from oil-packed to water-packed.

• If you like to snack, reach for plain, unbuttered popcorn instead of greasy potato chips.

• Keep cut-up vegetables in your refrigerator so they're always available to munch on. Carrots, green pepper, jicama, mushrooms and celery are all good choices.

• If you're craving a sweet, eat a piece of fruit or have a cup of herbal tea.

• Use no-stick pans to eliminate the need for oils and other fats when you fry or saute foods.

• Remove the skin from poultry before cooking.

• Steam vegetables and serve them with a squeeze of lemon.

• Use mozzarella cheese rather than cheddar or other high-fat cheeses.

• Eat meat only twice a week, substituting vegetables and salads.

• Drink plenty of water instead of sugary or artificially sweetened carbonated drinks.

• Eat ice milk or frozen yogurt instead of ice cream.

• Serve your meals on small, attractive dishes, bowls and plates.

• Eat low-fat rather than whole milk cottage cheese.

At a Restaurant

• Order your toast with the butter on the side; order your salads with the dressing on the side. That way you control the amount of fat that is added to your food.

• Order simple foods with a minimum of sauces, garnishes and toppings.

• Have a cup of coffee for dessert. Or have just a taste of a friend's dessert rather than ordering a full portion for yourself.

• If you love to nibble on bread, ask the person waiting on you to remove the basket of rolls from your table.

FOOD NUTRITION TABLE

Dairy Products

	Grams	Calories	Protein (gm)	Fat (gm)	Carbohydrates (gm)
Cheddar: Cut pieces (1 oz)	28	115	7	9	Trace
Mozzarella (whole milk) (1 oz)	28	90	6	7	1
Swiss cheese (1 oz)	28	105	8	8	1
Pasturized process cheese: American (1 oz)	28	105	6	9	Trace
Half-and-half (cream and milk) (1 cup)	242	315	7	28	10
Cream, sour (1 cup)	230	495	7	48	10
Whole milk (3.3% fat) (1 cup)	244	150	8	8	11
Low-fat milk (2%) (1 cup)	244	120	8	5	12
Nonfat milk (skim) (1 cup)	245	85	8	Trace	12
Buttermilk (1 cup)	245	100	8	2	12
Eggnog (commercial) (1 cup)	254	340	10	19	34
Shakes, chocolate (10.6 oz)	300	355	9	8	63
Ice cream (about 11% fat) (½ gal)	1064	2155	38	115	254
Ice cream (about 11% fat) (1 cup)	133	270	5	14	32
Ice milk: Hardened (about 4.3% fat) (½ gal)	1048	1470	41	45	232
Ice milk: Hardened (about 4.3% fat) (1 cup)	131	185	5	6	29
Tapioca (cooked) (1 cup)	260	320	9	8	59
Yogurt, fruit-flavored (8 oz)	227	230	10	3	42
Yogurt, plain (8 oz)	227	145	12	4	16

	Grams	Calories	Protein (gm)	Fat (gm)	Carbohydrates (gm)
Eggs					
Egg: whole, without shell (1 egg)	50	80	6	6	1
Egg, fried in butter	46	85	5	6	1
Scrambled (milk added) in butter. Also omelet.	64	95	6	7	1
Fats, Oils					
Butter, stick (½ cup)	113	815	1	92	Trace
Butter, tablespoon (about ⅛ stick)	14	100	Trace	12	Trace
Lard (1 cup)	205	1850	0	205	0
Margarine, stick (½ cup) (1 stick)	113	815	1	92	Trace
Corn oil (1 cup)	218	1925	0	218	0
Blue cheese, salad dressing (1 tbsp)	15	75	1	8	1
French dressing (1 tbsp)	16	65	Trace	6	3
Italian dressing (1 tbsp)	15	85	Trace	9	1
Fish, Shellfish, Meat, Poultry					
Clam, raw (3 oz)	85	65	11	1	—
Crabmeat (white or king), canned (1 cup)	135	135	24	3	0.1
Fish sticks, breaded, cooked. (1 fish stick)	28	50	5	3	—
Sardines, canned in oil (3 oz)	85	175	20	9	.5
Tuna, canned in oil, drained (3 oz)	85	170	24	7	.7
Bacon, 2 slices	15	85	4	8	.7
Ground beef, broiled, lean with 10% fat (3 oz)	85	185	23	10	.3
Steak, lean and fat (3 oz)	85	330	20	27	0
Beef and vegetable stew (1 cup)	245	220	16	11	15
Chili con carne with beans, canned (1 cup)	255	340	19	16	31
Chop suey with beef and pork (1 cup)	250	300	26	17	13
Liver, beef, fried (3 oz)	85	195	22	9	5
Luncheon meat (1 oz)	28	65	5	5	0
Bologna (1 slice)	28	85	3	8	Trace
Frankfurter (1 frankfurter)	56	170	7	15	1
Salami (1 slice)	10	45	2	4	Trace
Poultry and poultry products:					
Chicken, cooked, breast (2.8 oz)	79	160	26	5	1
Drumstick, fried (1.3 oz)	38	90	12	4	Trace
Chicken and noodles, cooked (1 cup)	240	365	22	18	26
Turkey, dark meat (4 pieces)	85	175	26	7	0
Turkey, light meat (2 pieces)	85	150	28	3	0
Fruits and Fruit Products					
Apple (1 apple)	138	80	Trace	1	20
Apple juice, bottled or canned (1 cup)	248	120	Trace	Trace	30
Applesauce, unsweetened (1 cup)	244	100	Trace	Trace	
Apricots, raw (3 apricots)	107	55	1	Trace	14
Avocados, California (1 avocado)	216	370	5	37	13
Banana (1 banana)	119	100	1	Trace	26
Blackberries (1 cup)	144	85	2	1	19
Cherries, sweet (10 cherries)	68	45	1	Trace	12
Dates, whole, without pits (10 dates)	80	220	2	Trace	58
Fruit cocktail, canned in syrup (1 cup)	255	195	1	Trace	50

	Grams	Calories	Protein (gm)	Fat (gm)	Carbohydrates (gm)
Grapefruit, pink or red (½ grapefruit with peel)	241	50	1	Trace	13
Grapes, Thompson seedless (10 grapes)	50	35	Trace	Trace	9
Grape drink, canned (1 cup)	250	135	Trace	Trace	35
Lemonade concentrate, frozen (6-fl oz can)	219	425	Trace	Trace	112
Lime juice, raw (1 cup)	246	65	1	Trace	22
Cantaloupe, (½ melon with rind)	477	80	2	Trace	20
Honeydew (1/10 melon with rind)	226	50	1	Trace	11
Orange (1 orange)	131	65	1	Trace	16
Orange juice, frozen concentrate (6-fl oz can)	213	360	5	Trace	87
Peach (1 peach)	100	40	1	Trace	10
Peach, dried, uncooked (1 cup)	160	420	5	1	109
Pear, Bartlett (1 pear)	164	100	1	1	25
Pineapple, raw, diced (1 cup)	155	80	1	Trace	21
Pineapple juice, unsweetened, canned (1 cup)	250	140	1	Trace	34
Plums, Japanese and hybrid (1 plum)	66	30	Trace	Trace	8
Prunes, uncooked (5 large prunes)	49	110	1	Trace	29
Raisins, seedless (1 cup)	145	420	4	Trace	112
Raspberries (1 cup)	123	70	1	1	17
Strawberries, frozen, sweetened (10 oz)	284	310	1	1	79
Tangerine (1 tangerine)	86	40	1	Trace	10

Grain Products

	Grams	Calories	Protein (gm)	Fat (gm)	Carbohydrates (gm)
Bagel, egg (1 bagel)	55	165	6	2	28
Biscuits, from home recipe (1 biscuit)	28	105	2	5	13
Cracked-wheat bread, loaf (1 lb)	454	1195	39	10	236
French bread, enriched (1 lb)	454	1315	41	14	251
Pumpernickel (1 lb)	454	1115	41	5	241
Whole-wheat bread (1 lb)	454	1095	41	12	4.2
Oatmeal or rolled oats cereal (1 cup)	240	130	5		1
Corn flakes, plain, added sugar, salt, iron, vitamins (1 cup)	25	95	2	Trace	21
Oats, puffed, added sugar, salt, minerals, vitamins (1 cup)	25	100	3	1	19
Rice, puffed, plain, added salt, iron, vitamins (1 cup)	15	60	1	Trace	13
Wheat flakes, added sugar, salt, iron, vitamins (1 cup)	30	105	3	Trace	24
Wheat, shredded, plain (1 biscuit)	25	90	2	1	20
Angelfood, whole cake (9¾-in. diam. tube cake)	635	1645	36	1	377
Cupcakes, with chocolate icing (1 cupcake)	36	130	2	5	21
Boston cream pie with custard filling, whole cake (8-in. diam.) (1 cake)	825	2490	41	78	412
Fruitcake (1 lb)	454	1720	22	69	271
Pound cake (1 slice)	33	160	2	10	16
Brownies (1 brownie)	20	95	1	6	10
Chocolate chip cookies, commercial, 2¼-in. diam., 3/8 in. thick (4 cookies)	42	200	2	9	29
Fig bars, square (1 5/8 by 1 5/8 by 3/8) (4 cookies)	56	200	2	3	42

	Grams	Calories	Protein (gm)	Fat (gm)	Carbohydrates (gm)
Oatmeal cookies with raisins, 2⅝-in. diam., ¼ in. thick	52	235	3	8	38
Vanilla wafers, 1¾-in. diam, ¼ in. thick (10 cookies)	40	185	2	6	30
Cornmeal, whole-ground, unbolted, dry (1 cup)	122	435	11	5	90
Graham crackers, 2½-in. square (2 crackers)	14	55	1	1	10
Doughnuts, cake type, plain, 2½-in. diam., high (1 doughnut)	25	100	1	5	13
Hot macaroni (1 cup)	140	155	5	1	32
Noodles (egg noodles), enriched, cooked (1 cup)	160	200	7	2	37
Noodles, chow mein, canned (1 cup)	45	220	6	11	26
Pancake, home recipe using enriched flour (1 cake)	27	60	2	2	9
Apple Pie (9-in. diam.) (1/7 of pie)	135	345	3	15	51
Cherry Pie (1/7 of pie)	135	350	4	15	52
Pecan Pie (1/7 of pie)	118	495	6	27	61
Pumpkin Pie (1/7 of pie)	130	275	5	15	32
Pizza (cheese) baked, 4¾-in. sector; ⅛ of 12-in. diam. pie (1 sector)	60	145	6	4	22
Popcorn, popped, plain, large kernel (1 cup)	6	25	1	Trace	5
Pretzels, 3¼ in by 2¼ in. by ¼ in. (10 pretzels)	60	235	6	3	46
Rice, white, enriched, instant, ready-to-serve, hot (1 cup)	165	180	4	Trace	40
Long grain rice, raw (1 cup)	185	670	12	1	149
Spaghetti, tender, served hot (1 cup)	140	155	5	1	32
Spaghetti (enriched) in tomato sauce with cheese (1 cup)	250	260	9	9	37
Waffles, 7-in. diam. (1 waffle)	75	210	7	7	28

Legumes (Dry), Nuts, Seeds

	Grams	Calories	Protein (gm)	Fat (gm)	Carbohydrates (gm)
Almonds, shelled, chopped (about 130 almonds) (1 cup)	130	775	24	70	25
Beans, dry, cooked, drained (1 cup)	180	210	14	1	36
Lima beans, cooked, drained (1 cup)	190	260	16	1	49
Blackeye peas, dry, cooked (1 cup)	250	190	13	1	35
Lentils, whole, cooked (1 cup)	200	210	16	Trace	39
Sunflower seeds, dry, hulled (1 cup)	145	810	35	69	29

Vegetable and Vegetable Products

	Grams	Calories	Protein (gm)	Fat (gm)	Carbohydrates (gm)
Asparagus, green, cooked, drained (1 cup)	145	30	3	Trace	5
Snap Beans, cooked, drained (1 cup)	125	30	2	Trace	7
Yellow Beans, cooked, drained (1 cup)	125	30	2	Trace	6
Bean sprouts (mung), raw (1 cup)	105	35	4	Trace	7
Beets, diced or sliced (1 cup)	170	55	2	Trace	12
Broccoli, cooked, drained, stalk, medium size	180	45	6	1	8
Frozen broccoli, stalk 4½ to 5 in. long	30	10	1	Trace	1
Brussels sprouts, cooked, drained (1 cup)	155	55	7	1	10

	Grams	Calories	Protein (gm)	Fat (gm)	Carbohydrates (gm)
Cabbage, raw, coarsely shredded or sliced (1 cup)	70	15	1	Trace	4
Carrots, whole, 7½ by 1⅛ in. (1 carrot)	72	30	1	Trace	7
Cauliflower, raw, chopped (1 cup)	115	31	3	Trace	6
Celery, stalk, large outer, 8 by 1½ (1 stalk)	40	5	Trace	Trace	2
Corn, sweet, cooked, drained (1 ear)	140	70	2	1	16
Lettuce, raw, 5-in. diam. (1 head)	220	25	2	Trace	4
Mushrooms, raw, sliced or chopped (1 cup)	70	20	2	Trace	3
Onions, raw, chopped (1 cup)	170	65	3	Trace	15
Peas, green, canned, whole, drained (1 cup)	170	150	8	1	29
Peas, frozen, cooked, drained (1 cup)	160	110	8	Trace	19
Potatoes, cooked, baked, peeled after baking (1 potato)	156	145	4	Trace	33
Potatoes, french-fried (10 strips)	50	135	2	7	18
Potato chips, 1¾ by 2½ in. oval cross section (10 chips)	20	115	1	8	10
Radishes, raw (prepackaged) stem ends, rootlets cut off	18	5	Trace	Trace	1
Spinach, raw, chopped, cooked, drained (1 cup)	55	15	2	Trace	2
Spinach, frozen, chopped (1 cup)	205	45	6	1	8
Tomatoes, raw 2⅗-in. diam. (1 tomato)	135	25	1	Trace	6
Miscellaneous Items					
Beer (12 fl. oz)	360	150	1	0	14
Wine, table (3½-fl. oz glass)	102	85	Trace	—	4
Root beer (12 fl. oz)	370	150	0	0	39
Olives, ripe (3 small or 2 large)	10	15	Trace	2	Trace
Soup, cream of chicken (with milk) (1 cup)	245	180	7	10	15

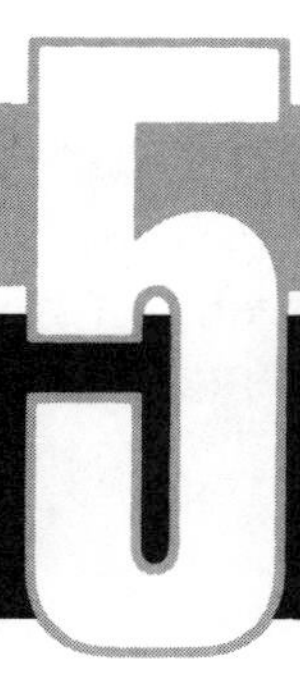

ROADBLOCKS TO IDEAL LEGS

The message from the moon . . . is that no problem need any longer be considered insoluble.

— *Norman Cousins*

Each of us has a flaw or two that keeps us from seeing ourselves as just the way we want to be. For many of us, our legs are our most difficult body part to keep in great shape. Some of the problems we encounter can be attributed to heredity, some to bad habits and some we can't seem to attribute to anything. But the most important step that we must take toward solving our problems (with our legs and with anything else in our lives) is to recognize them.

Remember our visualization exercises in the first chapter? That's where we focused on the good and the bad. Well, now, here's your chance to treat some of those problems that you may have with your legs. Focus on what you want to do, then do it. Don't forget to keep your fitness diary so that you can continue to chart your progress, especially in dealing with your leg problems.

CELLULITE

Quick now, what is lumpy, bumpy, seems to attach itself to the most unlikely places and is completely without socially redeeming value? If you answered cellulite, you're right. But wait just a minute — all the experts say there's no such thing, and so do the dictionaries. Then what's all the controversy about?

Back in 1973, Nicole Ronsard created a minor revolution when she published her book, *Cellulite: Those Lumps, Bumps and Bulges You Couldn't Lose Before.* The book detailed a six-part plan to aid you in the elimination of cellulite. Ronsard claimed that all you needed to do was to eliminate toxic wastes, adapt a natural diet and pay particular attention to your breathing and elimination habits, exercise, massage the affected areas and relax. Nonsense say the medical experts. As the AMA emphatically stated in 1976: "There is no medical condition known or described as cellulite in this country." The Medical Society of New York agrees, saying, "It is our opinion that books on cellulite exploit women through a gimmick . . . The truth is that fat is fat, and wherever it may be located in the body, it maintains its common characteristics."

That may be so, you say, but what about those lumps on the sides of my thighs? And how about the dimpled skin just above my knees when I pinch it. What do you call *that?*

As much as it might hurt to admit it, the so-called cellulite is just plain fat. It has its characteristic dimpled (some call it waffled or resembling cottage cheese) appearance because it's layer upon layer of irregularly distributed fat. Some call it "fat gone wrong," but it is actually a series of fat cells deposited immediately beneath the skin. The waffled appearance comes from the fibrous tissue strands that connect these fat cells to deeper tissue layers (including muscles) beneath the layers of fat. These tissue strands also connect to each other, creating a latticework effect.

Now that we've described the physical attributes of cellulite, the most important challenge is to learn how to deal with it. We've all seen those unattractive lumps of fat peeking out from under someone's shorts, or stuffed all too obviously into someone's too-tight jeans. How do we ensure that we will never fall victim to that lumpy, bumpy kind of fat? And if we have some, how do we get rid of it?

If you have cellulite, accept the fact that it is fat. It's an indicator that you're carrying more fat than your body can handle, and there's just no other place to conveniently deposit it. So because of our hormonal makeup, our female bodies tend to deposit these extra, irregularly shaped layers of fat in specific areas, which include the hips, thighs, breasts and buttocks. Men tend to deposit excess fat mostly around the abdomen — and they rarely tend to be affected by cellulite.

Since we now know that cellulite equals fat, we shouldn't succumb to advertising hype that offers miracle cures. Sorry, but no cream, no wrap treatments and no special massages will eliminate this fat. What it will take is dedication and commitment to burning it off. Exercises done for a specific area will help build and tone the underlying muscles, but they will not burn fat in that specific area. For example, if you do one hundred leg lifts, you will burn off some calories that will, in turn, burn fat — but that fat will not necessarily come from the exercised leg muscles.

But there is a solution. If you have cellulite, you very likely need to reduce your body's fat reserves, so from wherever you burn that fat, it's sure to be beneficial. Remember our old formula — it takes 3500 calories to burn one pound of fat. The best way to expend those calories is by reducing your caloric intake slightly, increasing your level of activity and reducing your fat intake. Aerobic exercise, particularly, will burn your excess fat. So refer to Chapter 6, on aerobic programs, to find one that you can stick with.

If you now have little dimpled knees or thighs, instead of blaming it on some insidious condition called cellulite, realize that it's just your body's way of telling you to get moving — so go to it.

SHINSPLINTS

Shinsplints is a painful condition resulting from a muscle imbalance between the calf and shin muscles. Typically, the calf muscles are much stronger than the shin muscles — so very logically, the best way to treat the condition is to strengthen the weaker shin muscles.

You'll know right away the symptoms of shinsplints; you'll feel tenderness in the front of your lower leg that is painful, hence the term "*shin*splints." This condition is often suffered by novice runners, but those who take aerobic dance classes can also develop the condition, because of the hard floors they often practice on.

As mentioned previously, the best way to treat shinsplints is to strengthen the shin muscle. This can be done by thoroughly warming up the lower leg with a series of stretching exercises. You can also strap a weight around your foot and exercise the calf by flexing the foot. This builds the outer calf muscles. Of course, if you are in good condition, you can rest or cut back on your running mileage until you're able to run pain-free again without getting out of shape. Or practice a sport that won't aggravate the condition, like swimming or cycling.

Other good preventive measures are to switch to a shoe with more padding and to exercise on a softer surface. If you currently run on a concrete sidewalk, switch to an asphalt street (asphalt is significantly softer than concrete); if you already run on a street, switch to running on dirt paths at the local park.

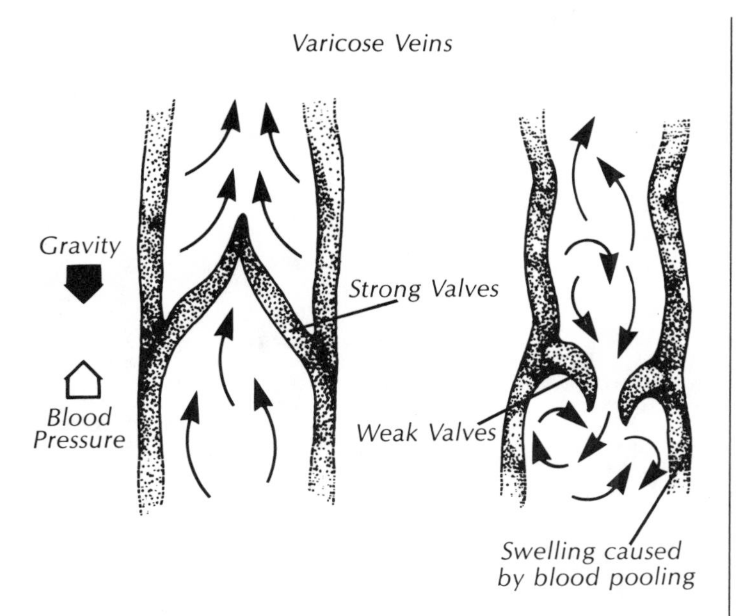

VARICOSE VEINS

If either your mom or your dad has varicose veins, chances are that you'll get them too. Don't blame them — it's a fact of genetics and heredity, just like your beautiful eye color and distinctive body type. You can't change what you have inherited, but you can certainly learn how to live with it.

Basically, varicose veins are swollen superficial veins. Since veins have valves in them that keep the blood traveling in one direction (toward the heart), one of the main causes of varicose veins is valves in the veins that leak. The blood flows backward or pools in the veins on the way back to the heart. The extra blood backing up in these veins weakens them and makes them thin from the swelling. The swollen condition is called varicose veins.

Certain conditions may aggravate or encourage the development of varicose veins. Obesity, pregnancy and the use of tight, constricting clothing, like girdles, definitely have an effect on their development. Obesity, by its very nature, stresses the body in any number of ways. It causes the development of swollen veins because of the added stress of carrying around fat. So for reasons other than appearance, if you're too heavy, lose that extra weight!

Pregnancy can create varicose veins, particularly in the latter months because of the inherent weight gain, and because of the increased blood flow to the abdominal area. Pregnant women are wise to avoid excessive weight gain because varicose veins can be an extremely uncomfortable addition to all the other pressures of pregnancy.

If you are afflicted with varicose veins or you suspect that you are a likely candidate to develop them, what should you do? First, don't worry about it; just learn what you can and then follow recommendations. Stay at your ideal weight. Participate in daily exercise that will benefit your leg circulation; running, bicycling, skating and swimming are all good. Avoid tight socks, stockings and even tight boots or shoes that might affect the circulation in your legs. However, good-fitting stockings can give some support to the varicose veins. Try not to cross your legs at the knees because that also affects the circulation. Avoid standing or sitting for long periods of time. Keep your legs elevated as much as possible to keep your blood from pooling.

The passive treatment techniques mentioned here should be all that today's woman who is active and fit-minded needs in dealing with varicose veins. But there are surgical and chemical injection treatments available, should you need them. Consult your doctor if you have a great deal of pain, or if you're concerned about the aesthetics of the condition.

SORE OR PULLED MUSCLES

The formula to remember when treating sore or pulled muscles is RICE, which stands for Rest, Ice, Compression and Elevation. Naturally, when you're injured you must give your body a chance to heal. That's where *rest* comes in; you'll know when it's time to start exercising again because your injury won't hurt.

Avoid the natural inclination to apply heat to your sore muscles right after the injury — that can prolong the healing time by causing more

Leg showing common injury sites.

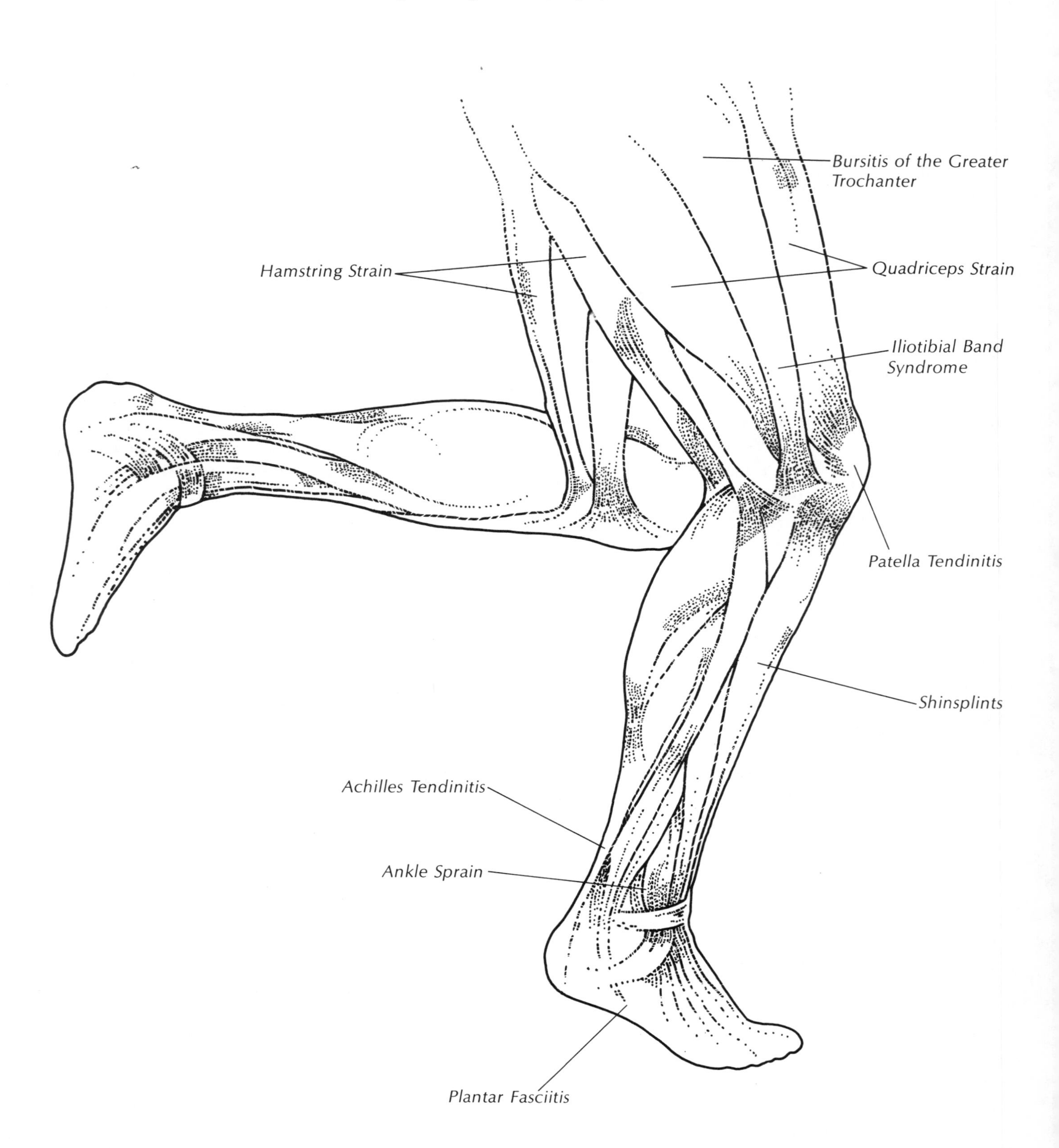

blood to flow to the injured area, resulting in congestion and more swelling. Instead, apply ice to the injury twice or even three times (about fifteen minutes per session) for the first two days following the injury. After two days you can switch to applying heat to the affected areas. Heating pads, soaks in a hot tub and analgesic creams such as Ben-Gay are all helpful at this stage of the injury.

Compression at the injury site reduces swelling. Wrap the affected area in an elastic bandage; be sure not to wrap it too tightly! Continue the compression treatment two or three times the first day of the injury.

Elevation helps to drain excess fluid from the injury, and reduces swelling. This can easily be accomplished by propping up your legs on a chair, table or even with pillows.

While injured, you may want to take plain or buffered aspirin. Aspirin is an effective anti-inflammatory agent that will contribute to the healing process. Remember that when you are injured, you must take care of your body to prevent further injury.

There's nothing more discouraging than having to sit out an event because of injury. Since you may not be used to participating in a regular fitness program, injury time is an easy time to give it up completely. Once you've followed the steps to treating an injury, just be determined to come back better than ever. Remember, you've made a commitment to yourself to have PRIDE: Personal Responsibility In Daily Effort.

OSTEOPOROSIS

Osteoporosis? Isn't that something old ladies get? If you think that, you're half right. The brittle bones of osteoporosis are typically suffered by post-menopausal women. Why are we also talking to young women about osteoporosis? Because according to a recent study at Oregon State University, exercise has a preventive effect on the development of osteoporosis.

What is osteoporosis? Basically, it's a condition of bone loss and deterioration caused by the depletion of calcium in the body. Brittle bones are easily fractured and are slow to heal. This is a problem suffered primarily by women — more than five million of them. Clearly, a condition that you want no part of.

The best way to prevent osteoporosis, it seems, is by supplementing your diet with calcium — ingesting plenty of dairy foods, especially milk, probably taking a calcium supplement (check with your doctor) and (what else?) regular periods of exercise to keep your bones strong. In the Oregon State University study, the bones of those age twenty to twenty-five were measured in relation to their activity levels. The high-activity group was found to have much denser bones that those of the low-activity group. Again, the message is — exercise for optimum health! Both for now and for when you get older. When classmates tease your grandchildren, saying, "Your grandma wears tennis shoes!" they can say, "That's right, and running shoes, and she bicycles and she's really healthy, too!"

MASSAGE FOR YOUR LEGS

After a tough workout, nothing feels better than a massage of your tired, aching muscles. The best experience would be at the hands of a professional. Your pains and aches will melt away; the cost is no more than the price of a haircut and shampoo — about $30 for one hour. If you're not comfortable with the idea of a professional massage, or you can't afford one, consider, instead, trading massages with a friend. Or, failing that, you can even give yourself a satisfying massage. Since a self-massage is a good way to learn technique, we'll give a few instructions. Once you know what feels good, you can be more confident about offering your services as a top-notch masseuse to other active friends.

The following is a series of suggested strokes you can try. The important point to remember when dealing with massage is to do what feels good; don't be afraid to apply pressure, and follow the contours of the body. Experiment and enjoy.

Think of dividing your leg into sections before you start your massage. Concentrate on one section at a time, massaging it thoroughly and completely before moving on to the next section. Treat the ankle, the lower leg and calf, the knee and the thighs as separate sections. You'll find that different techniques feel better on one section than another — make mental notes on the ones that you like best.

Ankle. The bony structure of the ankle necessitates small, circular movements here. Gently use your thumbs, rotating in circles to relax the ankle area. Use your body's contours to guide you — you'll know right away what feels good and what doesn't. When you're finished with the ankle, gently rotate it first one way, then the other, working out any lasting stresses you may feel.

Lower leg and calf. This area of your leg lends itself to long, deep stroking. Gently knead the muscles of your calf and use the same rotating thumb movements along your shin.

Knee. Your bony knee often gets sore since there are so many tendons and ligaments that hold everything in place here. Rotating your thumb in circles works well around the kneecap, as does some deep hand pressure just above the knee. Use your entire hand and all your fingers to cup your knee and stroke upward with your leg slightly bent. Don't try to massage the sensitive kneecap.

Thighs. The large area of your thigh lends itself to plenty of experimentation with different types of strokes. Use the heel of your hand on the front of your thigh and apply deep pressure, then gently knead the entire thigh. Next, stroke the area with your fingertips from knee to hip and then from side to side. Again, experiment until you find what feels just right. When you think you've mastered the art of self-massage, don't be shy about offering a muscle-relaxing massage to a friend. There's nothing like the exquisite sensation of touching and being touched. Follow your massage with a full-body relaxation exercise: Lie on your back and relax your entire body. As you relax let your mind run free and picture beautiful meadows, pristine mountain slopes covered with sparkling snow; warm sandy beaches in the sun — whatever suits your fancy at the moment.

HOW TO LIKE YOUR BODY BETTER

What do you do if you're on a program that keeps you at your ideal weight, you're healthy, active and feeling good, but you still don't like the body that Mother Nature has given you? Realize that you are your body; your personality and your body are inseparable and it's important that you come to terms with that concept. Love yourself, love your body — hate your body, hate yourself. It works both ways. How can you learn to love your body? Here are some tips:

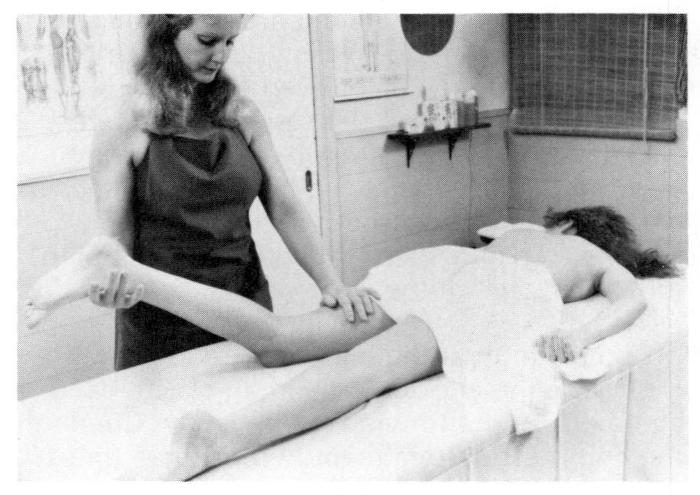

Massage is an ancient art still in use today.

1. Don't be a perfectionist. Realize that you'll never be perfect, but you can be excellent. Set reasonable rather than unattainable goals.

2. Learn to manage your time. Feeling comfortable with yourself necessitates that you have some sort of a regular schedule. Plan your weeks and your days so that you have time to exercise, time to reflect on your goals and time to assess your progress.

3. Learn more about diet and nutrition. Read a book or take a class on the subject. You may learn that you've been unwittingly subverting your efforts by improper food choices.

4. Learn to dress to flatter your figure. Notice the styles of clothing that look best on you. When your friends comment about how good you look, pay attention to the colors, fabrics and cut of your clothing. Why not wear what looks best on you?

5. Relax. Don't try to do too much. There are times in every person's life when it's appropriate to take a break and reflect. Where are you going and where have you been? Don't forget to have some fun along the way!

6 MOVING ON

The less of routine, the more of life.
— A. B. Alcott

The only way for you to burn fat and get your muscles in shape for good is to move your body. You must get off your duff and move! Lucky you, there are so many ways to get in shape.

You're not being fair to yourself when you use the excuse of no time to exercise. All it takes is an hour per day; you probably spend more time than that commuting to work, and certainly more time watching television. Think creatively and you can arrange the play time. If you really love to sit in front of the television, make it work for you — buy a stationary bicycle or a rebounder (a miniature trampoline) and spend a half-hour working up a sweat while watching your favorite sitcom. Rethink your priorities just a bit. If you usually stay up late, barely managing to get up and get going early in the morning, try something new. Force yourself to get to bed at a reasonable hour in order to wake up at six o'clock in the morning. Then convince yourself to go for a short run in the morning. It won't take long before you're hooked!

If you've led a sedentary life until now, it may be difficult to change some of your bad habits. Don't try to do it all at one time; you'll only increase your stress level in this already highly stressful world. Go easy on yourself, and learn to set reasonable goals that you know you can keep. For example, don't start running one week and then decide to enter a marathon in a month. Start running and plan to enter your first 5-K in two to three months. That's a reasonable goal, one that you can handle without too much stress.

WHY AEROBICS?

It seems that everything you read these days makes mention of aerobics — aerobic dance, aerobic fitness routines, aerobicise. What does all this mean and why all the fuss about aerobics anyway?

First, the Webster's dictionary definition of aerobic is, "able to live or grow only where free oxygen is present." So taken literally, of course, we are aerobic creatures who must have oxygen for survival. But the term "aerobic" has another definition, and while it is not yet recognized in any dictionary, it is just as important a concept as the first. The other definition of "aerobic" has to do with the quality of physical life. Ever since Ken Cooper coined the term back in 1968, (with his best-selling exercise book *Aerobics*) aerobics has been a means to an end for people interested in getting the most out of life. Basically, the second definition of aerobics relates to cardiovascular fitness. The efficiency of your heart and lungs and entire blood vessel system depends on your cardiovascular fitness and ability to exercise your body at its maximum level.

You've probably heard a great deal about how important it is to reach your target heart rate. If you participate in aerobic dance classes, the instructor may frequently stop the exercising and instruct you to find your heart rate. She may give you a mathematical formula that leaves you utterly confused and wondering just what is going on as everyone walks around with their hands on the sides of their necks, concentrating on their pulses. Well, you can and should be a part of that group. What's more, you can readily understand why reaching your target heart rate is important and learn to determine what yours is.

First, you must understand your resting heart rate, which is your heart rate when you are resting — that is, sitting down reading, watching television or enjoying a pleasant conversation. The typical American woman's resting heart rate is eighty beats per minute. The more fit your cardiovascular system, the lower your resting heart rate will be. It's not uncommon, for instance, to find that well-conditioned athletes have resting heart rates of forty to fifty beats per minute. I always feel a bit of pride when I give blood, because during the requisite blood pressure/pulse tests, the nurse invariably comments, "You're a runner, aren't you?" Even on as little as twenty to thirty miles per week, I manage to keep my resting pulse at about forty-eight.

A low heart rate is desirable during rest to give your body a chance to recuperate from stress. Theoretically, the fewer times your heart beats, the longer you can depend on your heart muscle to keep pumping. Let's look at two hypothetical people: Cathy, with a resting pulse of fifty and Karen with a resting pulse of eighty. At the end of just one hour, Cathy's heart has beaten 3000 times, but Karen's has beaten 4800 times. At the end of one twenty-four-hour period, Cathy's heart has beaten 72,000 times, but Karen's has beaten 115,200 times! Imagine the difference after five years, ten years!

Ironically, the only way to make your heart stonger and to lower your resting pulse is to force your body to work hard — to get your heart rate up and keep it there for a period of time. Your heart is a muscle, and like all muscles, the more you work it the stronger it becomes. And the secret to conditioning your heart is aerobic activity, any activity that increases your heart rate (to your target rate) and forces you to assimilate oxygen into your system. It should be sustained for a minimum of three times per week, twelve to twenty minutes per session.

Now, how do you determine your target heart rate? Partly, it's based on your age and your fitness level. Here goes:

1. Determine your resting heart rate. Rest your index and middle fingers on your neck until you find the pulse. Your finger is over the carotid artery, a major blood vessel that carries blood to the head. The pulse is easy to find here. Count the pulse for six seconds and multiply by ten. Take the pulse a few times and average the score for maximum accuracy.

2. Determine your maximum heart rate. This is a basic formula that is based on age; you should never exceed this heart rate because it could stress your heart. The formula is:

220 – your age = your maximum heart rate

3. Determine your target heart rate. Your target heart rate is 60 to 85 percent of your maximum heart rate, depending on your condition and intensity of workout. This is the level at which you should work out for the twelve to twenty minutes per day, at least three times per week in order to gain or maintain a minimum acceptable cardiovascular fitness.

Let's use our two hypothetical examples again: twenty-year-old Cathy, who's in great shape, and twenty-six-year-old Karen, who is out of shape and so needs to set her goals a bit lower.

Cathy

Resting Heart Rate = 50

Maximum Heart Rate = 200

(220 – 20 = 200)

Target Heart Rate = 170

(85% of 200)

Karen

Resting Heart Rate = 80

Maximum Heart Rate = 194

(220 – 26 = 194)

Target Heart Rate = 116

(60% of 194)

HEART RATE CHART

Age	Maximum Heart Rate (Beats per minute)	Exercise Heart Range (Beats per minute) 60%-85%
20 and below	200	120-170
21	199	119-169
22	198	119-168
23	197	118-168
24	196	117-167
25	195	117-166
26	194	116-165
27	193	115-164
28	192	114-164
29	191	114-163
30	190	113-162
31	189	112-161
32	188	112-160
33	187	111-159
34	186	110-158
35	185	110-157
36	184	109-156
37	183	108-156
38	182	107-155
39	181	107-154
40	180	106-153
41	179	105-152
42	178	105-151
43	177	104-151
44	176	103-150
45	175	103-149
46	174	102-158
47	173	101-147
48	172	100-146
49	171	100-145
50	170	109-145
51	169	108-144
52	168	108-143
53	167	107-142
54	166	106-141
55	165	106-140
56	164	105-139
57	163	104-139
58	162	103-138
59	161	103-137
60	160	102-136
61	159	101-135
62	158	101-134
63	157	100-134
64	156	99-133
65 and above	155	99-132

As you remember, Karen is not in as good shape as Cathy, so she should work up to her target heart rate slowly and deliberately, seeing it as a goal to reach. As you work yourself into better shape, you can gradually work your heart a little harder, thus increasing your cardiovascular strength and endurance. Naturally, it is advisable to see a physician before following the figures you see in the heart rate chart here showing target heart rates. It's important that you don't push yourself too hard or too fast, and that you work hard enough to obtain maximum benefits from each aerobic workout.

Many sportsmedicine clinics offer testing programs in which your target heart rate, your percentage of body fat and your blood chemistry levels can all be checked. If you're serious about improving your fitness level, you may want to participate in one of these programs. Often, universities, YMCAs and health clubs offer these programs, so they should be readily available wherever you live.

Other Aerobic Benefits

Now that you understand the cardiovascular benefits of aerobic sports, you will be pleased to know that there are other benefits from participating in aerobics — namely, burning fat. For every woman concerned about the size and shape of her legs and thighs, the issue of how to burn fat draws immediate and undivided attention. Fat is burned during aerobic activity. Since nearly every aerobic sport involves the use of the legs, the benefit is three-fold:

1. Cardiovascular
2. Fat burning
3. Building muscle strength

Clearly, aerobic workouts are beneficial. And if there is a history of heart disease in your family, it's very important to get your body and heart in shape. You'll be removing a significant risk of encountering heart trouble.

How do you find out which sports are for you? Trial and error is one way, but that can become expensive, and certainly time-consuming. Instead, evaluate your personality. Do you prefer to exercise with many people around? Or is it important to you to do your exercise

PLAY ACTIVITY	MINUTES TO BURN 100 CALORIES
Run/Jog (on flat)	9(5-15)
Climb stairs	10
Saw wood	10
Play racquetball	10
Swim	10(7-20)
Jump on trampoline	12
Mow lawn	12
Play soccer	13
Roller skate	15
Dance (aerobic)	15
Dig in garden	17
Cycle (on flat)	18(10-25)
Walk	20
Dance (disco)	20
Play table tennis	20
Play volleyball	20
Clean windows	20
Scrub floors	20
Rake leaves	20

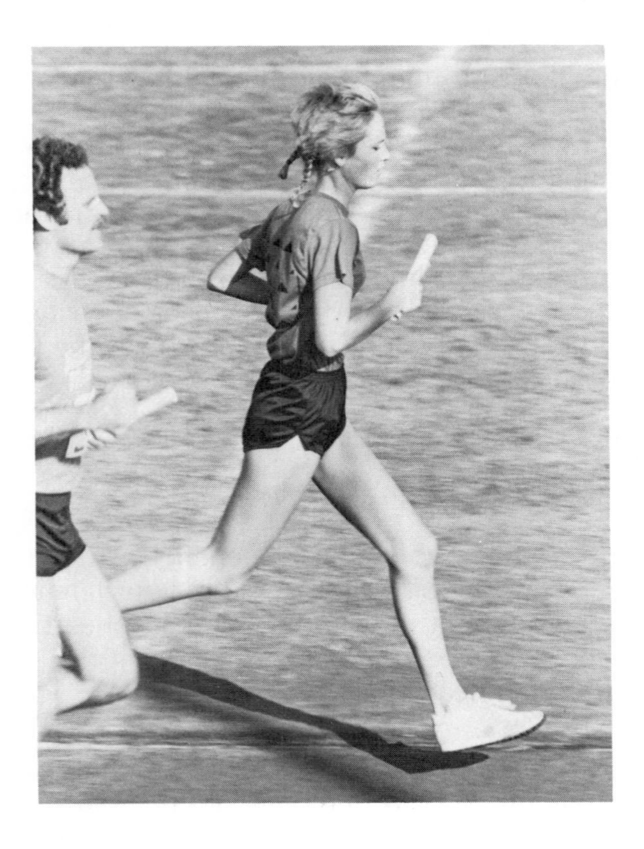

routine in private? Do you prefer team or individual sports? Do you enjoy playing inside or outside?

After you answer those questions, think about your body and how you respond to certain situations. Are you fairly strong, flexible and quick on your feet? Are you well coordinated or clumsy? How strong are your arms? your legs?

Another consideration is money. Do you have a six-figure income that allows you to join a trendy health club? What about joining a less expensive club? Or do you need to be in a health club at all? Some sports require special equipment that can be expensive. Other sports, like running, require only good shoes.

Presumably you've spent some time thinking about the sports you want to pursue in order to develop and maintain fitness. The following list of the best, most popular aerobic sports may help you choose a sport if you still haven't decided. Since this publication is primarily concerned with shaping up the legs and thighs, we've picked sports that are particularly good for them.

RUNNING

Taking up running can be one of the most liberating decisions of your life. There's an incredibly free, exhilarating feeling when you take to the streets. That youthful energy you once had is rediscovered. Remember how good it felt to run races against the neighborhood kids when you were young? To play tag or hide-and-seek? That same joy will reawaken when you pursue running as a fitness sport.

One of the finer characteristics of the sport is the ease with which you can chart your progress. When you start, you may have difficulty completing just a quarter-mile. But soon you'll notice that you feel strong enough to go twice that distance, then three, four, even twelve times the original distance. Where else in your life can you see that kind of dramatic improvement in your performance? Thirty million Americans (who run regularly) can't be wrong — they subscribe to at least three magazines on the subject and read a phenomenal number of books on the sport, ranging from running for women to Zen and the art of running. That's quite a cross section! What is it that these runners find so appealing?

First, running can be a downright cheap sport — all you need is a good pair of shoes. Your shorts, shirts, sweats and socks can easily be borrowed from your casual-wear wardrobe. Another advantage of running is that you can do it practically anywhere. Off on a business trip? Going to the park? Wherever you are, it's no problem to lace up your shoes, open the door and start out on a new adventure. There are very few sports that require so little equipment.

Additionally, running can be enjoyed on many different levels. You can easily start a running program, even if you have been sedentary for years. Of course, if you've been inactive for many years, it's always wise to have a physical examination by your doctor before beginning any exercise program. Start at your own pace — whatever feels comfortable. The idea at first isn't to race, but to *move* that body. If you're embarrassed by your lack of speed, all the more reason to keep going. Running is just like any other skill; the more you practice, the better you become. You might prefer to run with another person who's at the same level of expertise as yourself. The "buddy" system may help you to stay motivated and to keep going when otherwise you might stop. Running with a friend also helps you learn to pace. You should be able to carry on a conversation as you run; if you get winded, you're running too fast.

Once you feel comfortable lacing up those good running shoes and working out regularly, you will very likely start looking for a new challenge. You might explore the nearby countryside on challenging running trails, you might want to learn to increase your speed and/or distance, or you might decide to start running races. Fun-runs, 5- and 10-K races, half- and full marathons have become a part of the American scene. Running a race is certainly a challenge, both mentally and physically. It will allow you the opportunity to compare your speed and style with hundreds of other runners. More importantly, you'll be able to learn your limits: your threshold of pain, your stamina and desire. You'll meet interesting, fun-loving people who share the common interest of physical fitness and the active life and, what's more, you'll be having fun.

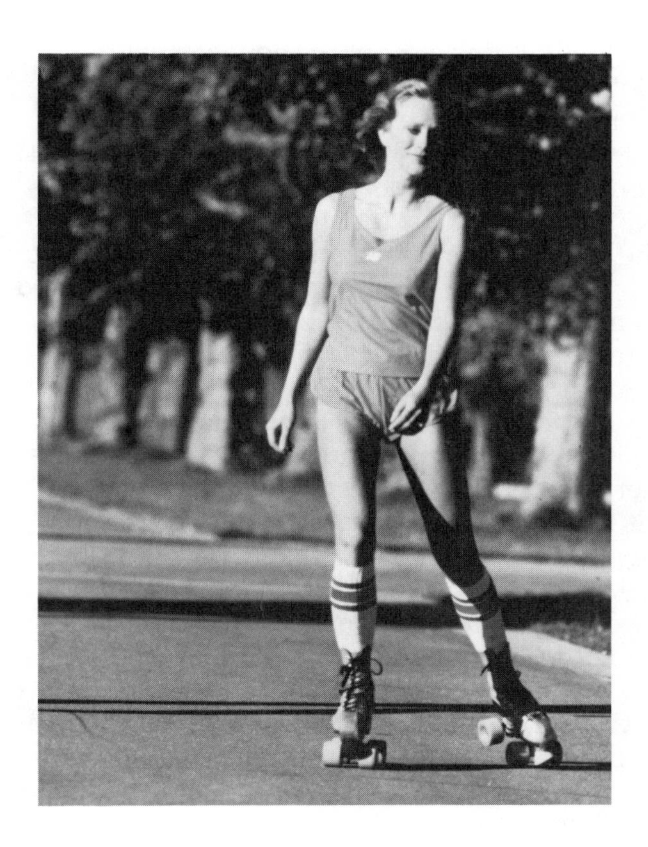

Besides the obvious cardiovascular benefits gained from running, it is a good workout for your legs and thighs. If you think of running in terms of repetition of a certain movement, consider all the times you raise your legs on a short, one-mile run. Running also increases your leg strength. If you need further proof, notice the strong and powerful legs and thighs of the women you see gathered at the next local 10-K.

ROLLER SKATING

The sport of roller skating has been around since the 1800s, enjoying varying degrees of popularity ever since. The most recent roller skating boom, in the late 1970s, led to a number of scientific inquiries about the benefits of the sport. When we call roller skating a sport, we're not talking about merely cruising around the rink all decked out in the latest glitter clothing. We are suggesting a whole-body workout of considerable value. In 1981, Dr. Allen Selner, a noted sportsmedicine podiatrist, conducted (in cooperation with the sports department at UCLA) a comprehensive study of the benefits of roller skating as an aerobic activity. Selner's testing program has been reported in a number of medical journals and general interest publications.

He found that after a ten-week program of roller skating thirty minutes per day, five days per week, his test subjects reduced their body fat levels an average of 4.2 percent, gained significantly in leg strength (23 percent), increased their maximum oxygen consumption levels by 17 percent and lowered their blood cholesterol levels by 6.3 percent.

Other benefits of roller skating for your legs and thighs are obvious to the casual observer at any roller skating center. There's not a speck of "cellulite" to be seen on any roller skating enthusiast who glides around the floor wearing the skimpiest of outfits. Roller skating effectively works all the muscles in the thighs — trouble spots for so many women. The sleek thighs of roller skating champions like Anna Conklin and Sandy Dulaney give silent testimonial to that fact.

For people with joint problems or who are severely overweight, roller skating can be a practical alternative to running as an aerobic sport. The gliding motion of skating eliminates much of the pounding and stress on the knees, which can be a problem for some runners. And roller skating can seem like an effortless way to exercise — it can be used as an effective form of transportation, you can enjoy it alone or very socially with many friends. You can even participate (at least indoors) morning, noon or night — in any kind of weather — at your local skating center.

Many roller skating centers have introduced aerobic roller skating classes, and if competition is in your blood, you might even want to join a competitive speed team for the workout of your life. If you were an enthusiastic roller disco skater a few years ago, rethink the possibilities your stored skates can still offer you.

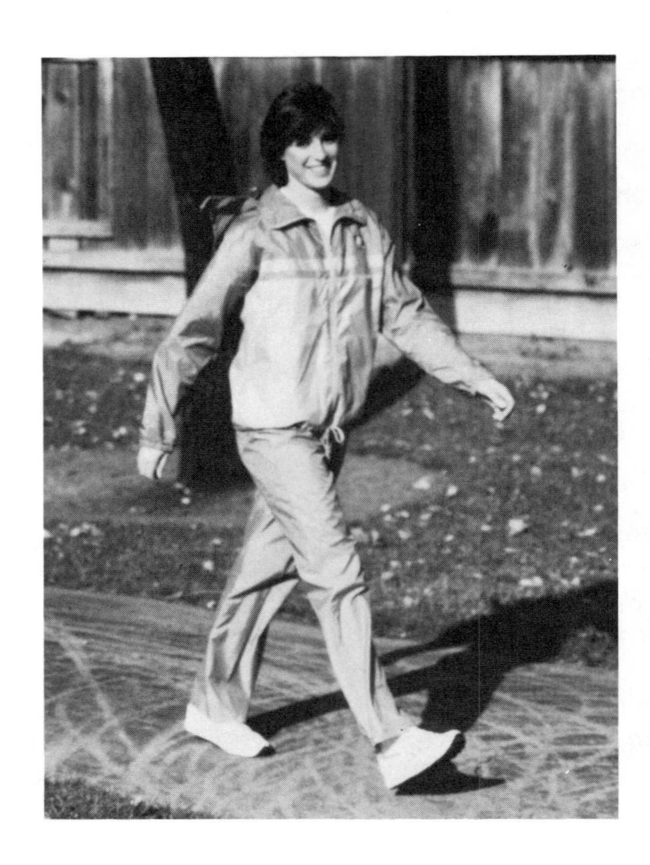

WALKING

Walking is perhaps the easiest and least expensive way to get and keep your legs and thighs in shape, but also the most time-consuming. However, you can fit a walk into your schedule, especially if you decide to walk to work, to the bus stop or perhaps during your lunch break. You can move along at a pretty fast clip (three to five miles per hour) while walking. It's fun, too, to take up a walking plan with a friend. You can easily carry on a conversation while walking at a speed that's burning about one hundred calories per mile.

The secret to walking your way to fitness is to get your heart rate up and to keep it there for twenty to thirty minutes per session. Consistency is also important; you must walk a minimum of three days per week to keep your present level of fitness, and more to increase it.

A good way to start a running program is by walking. You may find it more comfortable at first to alternate walking with jogging, until you feel comfortable with running.

All you need for walking is a good pair of comfortable running shoes. You can even wear your running (walking) shoes with a dress or suit and carry your dress shoes as you walk to work. Or if you must drive or rely on public transportation, either park a little farther from your office or get off at an earlier stop in order to give yourself a longer walk in the morning and the evening. There's no better way to start or finish a hectic, stress-filled day than with a little exercise.

Walking provides your legs and thighs with the same type of workout that you can get from running, but it eliminates much of the stress. Many people don't like to run, but they think that it's the only way to stay in shape. Walking may not work as quickly, but in time you can strengthen your leg muscles and upgrade your cardiovascular system almost as well as if you were running. Walking tends to work your thigh and calf muscles equally, which reduces the chance of injury from a muscle imbalance.

DANCING

Dancing is one of the most universal of movements. Every culture celebrates the joy of movement set to music, in one way or another. Whether you enjoy the highly structured, classical movements and positions in ballet or the free-flowing beauty of modern dance, or even the fun of pogoing on a New Wave dance floor, dance is movement, and movement burns calories.

One reason why dancing is so good for your legs and thighs is because it involves repetition of select movements. You often will stay in the bent-knee position when on the dance floor — a position that's particularly effective in strengthening and slimming the thighs.

Another beauty of dance is the opportunity you have to express yourself. Have you ever experienced the sheer joy of tuning in to your favorite radio station and moving spontaneously to the music? If you haven't, try it. It can be a lot of fun.

If you prefer more structure in your dancing, consider taking a ballet or jazz class at your

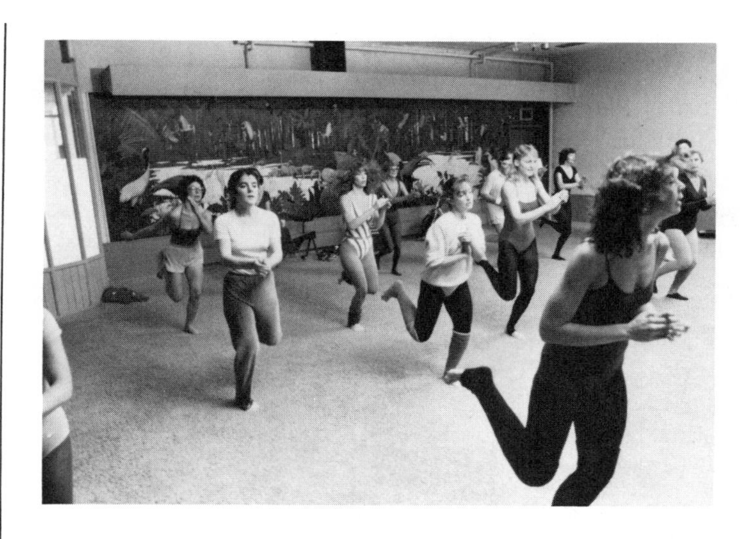

local YWCA, or at a nearby community college. You'll find that the discipline of regular classes will have a positive effect. Dancing will also increase your balance and gracefulness, which is another plus.

Aerobic Dancing

A highly structured dance activity that might appeal to you is aerobic dancing. There are any number of different manifestations of this form of exercise: Jazzercise, Dancercise, Dance Energetics and Aerobic Dance are just a few. You might take a few different types of classes before you settle on any one. But any good aerobic dance workout should include a warm-up of no less than five minutes, a twenty-minute aerobic routine, a stretching period and a good cooldown. Many instructors will also encourage you to count your heart rate at different times during the routine. Do it. It's a good way to find out if you're getting enough benefit from your workout. You should work up a sweat during a good dance workout, so dress accordingly; a leotard and tights are the most comfortable, particularly if they are made of cotton, which helps absorb perspiration.

When starting a dance class, do your best to keep up with the rest of the class, but don't hesitate to stop if you're feeling winded, lightheaded or in any way uncomfortable or dizzy. And to protect your knees and the muscles in your shins and calves, try to exercise on a padded mat, or at least on carpet; the padding will reduce stress to your leg muscles. Remember to have fun. Exercising to music should be pleasurable.

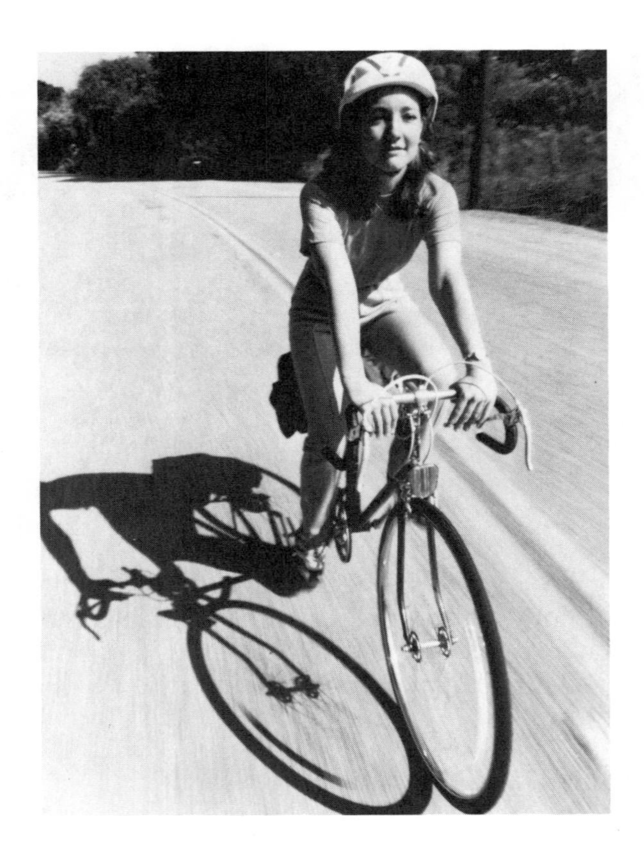

BICYCLING

Remember the old saying, "Once you learn how to ride a bicycle, you'll never forget." It's probably true. But as entrepreneur and triathlete Sally Edwards says in her book, *Triathlon: A Triple-Fitness Sport,* "Cycling is a sport of extremes: simple to learn, yet difficult to master; easier than walking at slow speeds, yet totally exhausting at full power; physically simple, yet mechanically complex."

You can use cycling as a means to get around town, as a pleasant way to spend a social afternoon or, on a more intense level, you can use bicycling as your training method. Bicycling is a good sport for keeping your legs, particularly your thighs, in great shape. Few sports can work your leg muscles so intensely with such quick trimming results. The smooth, repetitive movement of cycling is what makes it an effective way to trim your legs. The workout you get from bicycling, of course, depends on what you put into it.

The quality of your bicycle does, to some extent, determine how far, how fast and how intensely you can ride comfortably. For that reason, and for safety, your bicycle should be of the highest quality you can afford. Visit your local bicycle shop and ask for help in picking the right bike for you. The salesperson will be able to help you find the proper size frame.

Safety Products and Clothing

Once you've purchased your bicycle, why not give some consideration to safety? Since you'll be bicycling on city streets and dealing with traffic and a variety of other road hazards, a helmet is a must. Good helmets cost between $35 and $50. Also, learn the rules of the road and how to ride your bike. Other safety gear includes cycling gloves. They protect your hands in case of a fall and provide padding to protect the sensitive nerves in your hands. You should also attach a water bottle/cage to your bicycle, being sure to drink regularly to avoid dehydration.

The best type of clothing for bicycling is found at bike shops. Snug-fitting jerseys with pockets and chamois-lined shorts are both comfortable and functional. Jerseys look nice and reduce wind resistance because of their tailored fit. Bicycling shoes with cleats that fit into the pedal with toe clips are preferred by some; but stiff-soled touring shoes without the cleats are just as comfortable and easier to walk around in.

Learning to Ride

When learning to cycle properly, try not to "burn yourself out." Many novice women riders will attempt to keep up with a more experienced rider, but quickly realize that they do not have the strength to keep up. Don't get discouraged, though. Maybe you are using the wrong gears on your ten-speed. Even if you are as strong as the experienced rider, through proper gear selection she will have a big advantage. Familiarize yourself with cycling terminology and gearing by joining a bike club, and reading up on the sport.

Bicycling burns calories and tones the leg muscles almost as efficiently as running. If you need further proof, look in a bicycle magazine at the legs of top female cyclists who are training for the 1984 Olympics. Rebecca Twigg and

Jacque Bradley, riding for the Southland Corporation team, are two young standouts in super shape. And the strong and powerful legs of both Beth Heiden, Connie Carpenter and Sarah Docter have captured the imaginations of cycling and physical fitness buffs at the popular Coors Classic bicycle races in Colorado.

The fundamental rule to effective cycling for trimming and toning your legs is in maintaining proper cadence (turning of the pedals). Learn how to arrange your gears so that you pedal within a suitable range, say sixty to ninety rpm. Too many beginners think that it has to hurt to be effective; they end up pushing very hard gears (big ones) and risk injuring their knees. When you ride up hills, you should learn to shift into a low gear that will enable you to keep up a steady cadence. If you fear using your gears, there is no point in owning a ten-speed. And it's no fun having to get off and push your bicycle halfway up a hill. That's not the point of owning a bike. Learn to ride it up hills. Riding up hills offers the advantage of being valuable for working out your thighs, too.

When your thighs are hurting, after a hard climb for example, the worst is over. The burning sensation you might experience results from a buildup of lactic acid in the muscles. It means that you are exercising so hard that your body can't keep up. Once you start coasting down the hill, your legs will have a chance to recover and you can continue your ride pain-free.

Although we have outlined only the best exercises for your legs and thighs, you may have other interests. Some sports that are beneficial for strengthening and toning your legs include tennis, cross-country skiing, soccer and swimming.

Tennis

While tennis isn't particularly beneficial for losing weight (because it's not an aerobic sport in the strictest sense), the fact that you're on your feet and on the move can be very good for strengthening your legs. Your muscles will be used in many different ways as you change directions on the court, allowing more of a workout for all the muscles. Tennis can, however, be hard on your knees because of all the stopping and starting and sudden twisting motions common to playing.

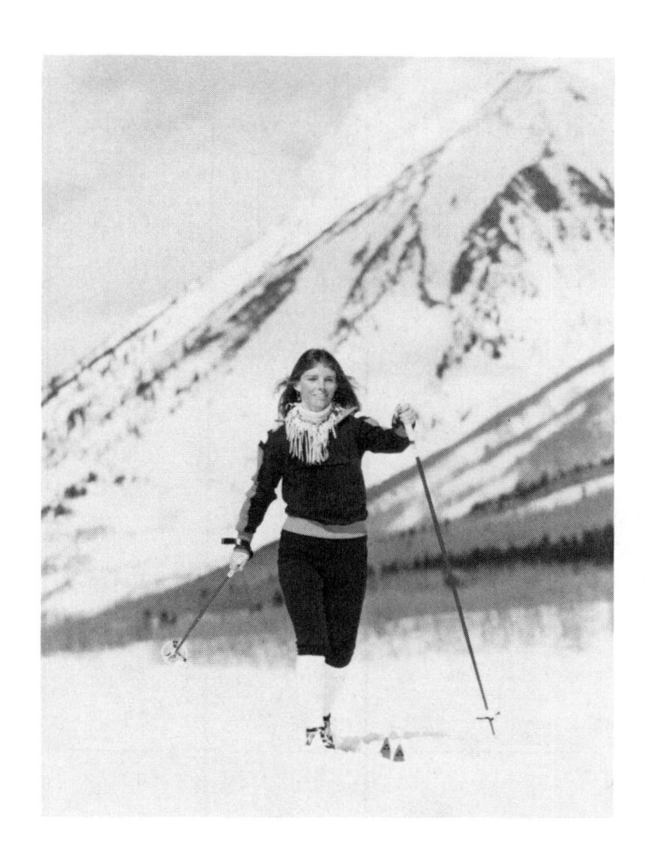

Cross-Country Skiing

Cross-country skiing, by its very nature, is not available to much of the population for a large part of the year. But if you have the opportunity, give both cross-country and downhill skiing a try. Neither one of these sports should be attempted unless you're in good shape. Both are demanding and require a considerable amount of strength, concentration, coordination and endurance.

Team Sports

Soccer and other team sports like field hockey, lacrosse and basketball are good strength-building sports for women. These sports rely primarily on running for exercise, but it's not as steady as with jogging, so it is not quite as good for aerobic conditioning. Participation in team sports is a way of making friends with similar interests.

Swimming

Swimming is an all-around conditioning exercise that also offers suitable aerobic benefits

RATING FOURTEEN POPULAR SPORTS

Physical Fitness	Running/ Jogging	Bicycling	Swimming	Skating (Ice or Roller)	Handball/ Squash	Skiing-Nordic (Cross-Country)	Basketball
Cardiorespiratory endurance (stamina)	21	19	21	18	19	19	19
Muscular endurance	20	18	20	17	18	19	17
Muscular strength	17	16	14	15	15	15	15
Flexibility	9	9	15	13	16	14	13
Balance	17	18	12	20	17	16	16
General Well-Being							
Weight control	21	20	15	17	19	17	19
Muscle definition	14	15	14	14	11	12	13
Digestion	13	12	13	11	13	12	10
Sleep	16	15	16	15	12	15	12
Total	148	142	140	140	140	139	134

Physical Fitness	Skiing-Alpine (Down-hill)	Tennis	Calisthenics (Aerobic Dancing)	Walking	Golf (with cart or caddy)	Softball	Bowling
Cardiorespiratory endurance (stamina)	16	16	10	13	8	6	5
Muscular endurance	18	16	13	14	8	8	5
Muscular strength	15	14	16	11	9	7	5
Flexibility	14	14	19	7	8	9	7
Balance	21	16	15	8	8	7	6
General Well-Being							
Weight control	15	16	12	13	6	7	5
Muscle definition	14	13	18	11	6	5	5
Digestion	9	12	11	11	7	8	7
Sleep	12	11	12	14	6	7	6
Total	134	128	126	102	66	64	51

Adapted from Conrad C. Carson, "How Different Sports Rate in Producing Physical Fitness," President's Council on Physical Fitness and Sports, Washington, D.C., U.S. Department of Health, Education and Welfare, Public Health Service, February 1979. These ratings were computed by averaging the ratings given each sport and exercise by seven physical fitness experts.

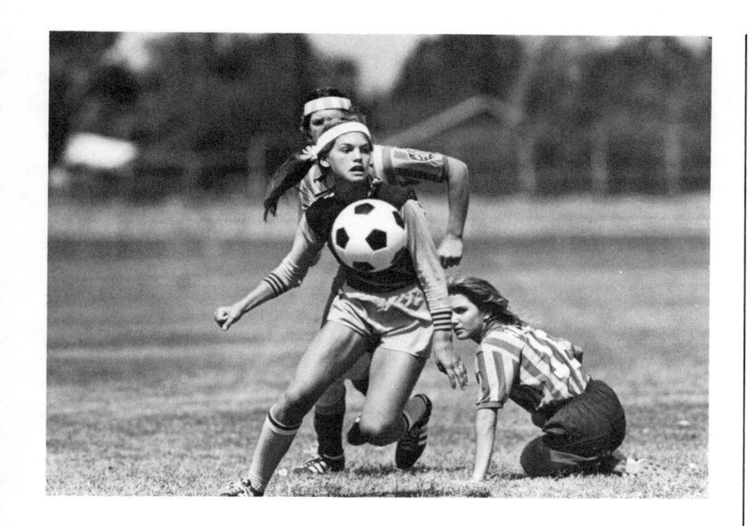

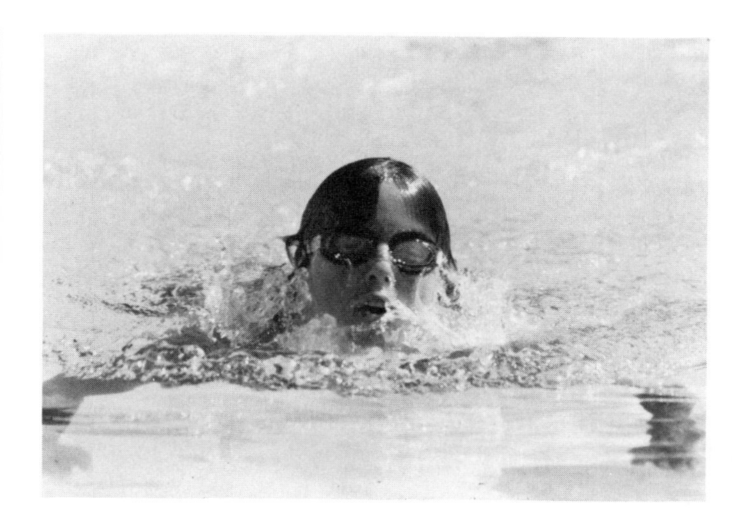

that are of value. It is not joint-stressful. The buoyancy provided by water removes weight from the joints and muscles, yet it does not hinder you from getting in a good workout. Swimming is an ideal alternative to other aerobic sports, especially if you're nursing an injury or just want a break from your regular routine. If you've always been a recreational swimmer and want to learn how to improve your stroke and become more efficient at breathing, you should take a swimming course. Consult a nearby junior college, recreation center or join a masters' swim program at your local YWCA.

All you'll need to swim is a tank suit, goggles, bathing cap and a good shower after your workout; the high level of chlorine in swimming pools can cause your skin and hair to lose their natural oils, so take that shower.

COMPARATIVE COSTS OF LEG-STRENGTHENING ACTIVITIES

Running. Running shoes will cost anywhere from $30 to $100. A very good pair of shoes can be bought for less than $50. Shorts, T-shirts and sweatshirts are probably already in your wardrobe, so there's no need to purchase special running clothing. If you do, plan on spending $100.

Roller Skating. Skates will cost upwards from $75. Look for quality leather boots; sealed precision bearings and urethane wheels. You may want to purchase safety equipment for outdoor use (knee guards, wrist guards and/or elbow pads). Rink costs are usually less than $4 for a two- to four-hour session.

Walking. All you need for walking is a good, sturdy pair of walking or running shoes (see above).

Bicycling. A satisfactory exercise ten-speed bicycle that will allow you to commute and ride comfortably in excess of fifty miles will cost anywhere from $250 to $300. Don't buy the cheap $90 ten-speeds; they fall apart quickly and spare parts are impossible to purchase. Most bicycle mechanics refuse to work on them.

Dancing. Cost varies, starting at no charge and going as high as you like. One way to try aerobic dance is to purchase an aerobic-dance exercise record. Or watch the newspapers for special offers at dance classes. Club memberships often are $30 to $50 a month.

7 WOMEN MUSCLE IN

Since magazines both set the style and reflect our society's values, you had to get the feeling that a change was in the wind when a popular, mainstream magazine like *Life* featured a cover story on women who lift weights to keep in shape. No off-the-wall, body-building publication — this photo-feature magazine has been in business for decades. The story was entitled, "Women Discover the Joy of Pecs — and Lats and Abs," and it documented, in the October 1982 issue, the joys that women are discovering through shaping their bodies by weight training.

Barbells, Nautilus and Universal gyms are no longer considered off-limits to the female athlete. This is certainly a change from as recently as 1964, when Olympian Wyomia Tyus said, "Our runners don't lift any weights because they're afraid of getting muscles." Today's woman simply is not afraid of getting "muscles." In fact, the muscled, well-defined body is the new ideal. Women today admire the strong and well-toned bodies of such popular actresses as Victoria Principal and Jane Fonda; the strength of athletes like Martina Navratilova and Grete Waitz, and the fitness of older notables like Raquel Welch and Linda Evans. These strong role models definitely reflect the new status that today's woman has in Western society. In essence, we have become physically stronger because we've been perceived as more competent, and more capable.

WHY WEIGHTS?

Why do women train with weights? The answers vary, but many women discover that weight training affords them the first real strength and power they've ever experienced. Working with weights tones, conditions and strengthens muscles like no other activity. And beyond the physical benefits, weight training is fun. You see almost immediate results. You can streamline the shape of your body, you can increase bulk and you can decrease body fat by training with weights. As you learn more about your body, you can actually shape it to look its absolute best through weight training. Says Arnold Schwarzenegger, "Once you see your body changing, you feel a sense of achievement and confidence. That, in turn, starts the mind believing it can do more and more. From there, the possibilities are almost limitless." And body builder Rachel McLish adds, "You have a simple choice of what to put on your bones: fat or muscle. Working out is a positive addiction."

You should remember that weight training can also bulk up the muscles in women. (Although not to the degree that it can with men, because women have insufficient male hormones.) Many women, in their zeal to pursue and excel in the enjoyment of weight training, begin by lifting as much weight as they can, as fast as they can. If you're interested in adding bulk, that may be okay, but you need to be aware that you can very easily and quickly add inches to your body without meaning to. Spend a little time, therefore, planning your weight training goals so that you don't spend unneeded energy creating what you don't want. The other possibility to consider is that there may be areas, your calves for instance, where you will want to add muscle. Once you're clear about your goals, talk to a weight trainer or consult a weight training book for the type of program that you should undertake.

Some women become so thrilled with the changes in their bodies when they begin to lift weights that they just keep adding weight — and adding inches. So take it slow and easy, and be sure to record each session so that you have a point of reference. Most health clubs with weight training facilities have a workout chart available — or you can easily create your own by following the example here.

Date	Exercise	Sets and Repetitions	Weight
2/2	Hamstring Machine	2 sets of 20	20 lbs.
2/2	Quad Machine	2 sets of 20	10 lbs.
2/2	Cable Machine	1 set of 12	10 lbs.

Give your muscles a chance to rest at least one full day between weight training sessions. A good schedule would be to work out in the weight room on Monday, Wednesday and Friday. You could pursue an aerobic conditioning program on your days off.

Stretching should be an integral part of your weight training program; it will help to keep the muscles loose and help you recover more comfortably from the workout. Spend ten to fifteen minutes stretching, minimum, before and after lifting weights. See Chapter 8 for special stretching routines.

In your weight training, as with all other projects in your life, remember that no one plan works for everyone. Vary your routine from time to time, if for no other reason than to guarantee that you do not become bored with it. Be kind to yourself; don't be afraid to schedule a day off or even to skip a day if you're not feeling up to par. The old cliche is that all work and no play makes Jack (or Jill) a dull boy (or girl). Don't allow your play to become work — just work hard at it, but enjoy it at the same time.

Weight Training Terminology

Exhaustion — The point at which the muscle can no longer perform a desired movement.

Repetitions — One complete movement of a specific exercise.

Resistance — Amount of weight.

Set — The number of repetitions performed in succession, usually with a rest period in between.

WHERE TO WORK OUT

It's not necessary to join a club to work out with weights, but you may find it beneficial because the staff members usually are well informed about how to work with weights in order to achieve the results you want. They know what routines you should follow, how many repetitions (reps) to do and how much weight you should use in order to sculpt and tone your body. When you're starting out, it is a good idea to consult with an expert. You may also find that joining a health club helps you stay motivated, especially when you consider that it usually involves an initial outlay of cash.

The atmosphere in most health clubs is fitness-oriented — the patrons are there to get in shape, and most members of a good club with a weight training program will be more than willing to give you assistance with the unfamiliar routines. Health clubs often have a social calendar, which will give you opportunities to make new, fitness-oriented friendships. You may live at a condominium or apartment complex where you have access to weight training equipment, or the company where you work or the school you attend may have a weight room for you to use. Investigate the possibilities and remember, too, that it is possible to train with weights at home. You'll need to purchase specialized equipment — free weights, a good bench and support system.

WHAT TO LOOK FOR IN A HEALTH CLUB

If you decide to take up weight training, you might want to join a health club. It's often impractical to do a great deal of weight training at home, so unless you live at an apartment or condominium complex where you have access to a weight room, you'll have to think about joining a club that offers Universal, Nautilus, free weights or a combination of the three.

Your first consideration when contemplating joining a club is cost. Payments can vary from an annual assessment to a monthly installment plan for five years, or longer. Be prepared, if you decide to visit a "spa," to listen to the sales pitch of the attendant. Many of these employee/salespeople work on commission, so they might make promises of services that are nonexistent, just so that they can "close the deal." So have a list of what it is that you want when you go into a health club. Be certain that the types of facilities you want are available to you, and don't be swayed by high-pressure sales techniques designed to dupe you into signing a contract that you may or may not want.

Some points to consider:

1. Check the club for cleanliness: the locker room, the floors in the exercise area, the showers, the obscure corners of the club. Are they clean enough for your standards?

2. Visit the club during peak hours (usually 5 p.m. to 7 p.m.) and again during off-hours. Take a look at the people who are working out — do they appear to be the type of people that you want to spend your time with? Are there long lines at each weight station? If your intention is just to get in, work out and then leave, you might want a large club that offers many different types of machines, or you may be able to schedule your training around the club's peak hours.

3. Does the club offer a number of facilities that seem desirable to you? If the club has tennis and racquetball courts, but you dislike racket sports, it may not be the best place for you. Make sure that the club you join offers just what you want; remember that you'll still be paying for all the fancy extras whether you use them or not. On the other hand, maybe the idea of learning a new sport or taking advantage of the Jacuzzi and whirlpool, saunas and steam baths appeals to you. You be the judge.

4. Is the atmosphere healthy? That is, find out the club's policy on smoking in the facility. And find out if there is a juice bar or area where you can purchase healthy refreshments after a tough workout.

5. What types of qualifications does the staff have? Many clubs offer the services of exercise physiologists, physical therapists, nutritionists and other professionals in the health care field. Other clubs may not have such a well-trained staff. Again, it's up to you to determine what's important.

6. What is the social atmosphere of the club and how does it compare with what you want? Many fitness centers seem to be the 1980s version of the singles bar of the 1970s. Many offer "get acquainted" potlucks and happy hours. These activities may appeal to you as a great place in which you can meet friends who have interests similar to your own. Or you may not want to associate with the people you work out with; it's all a matter of personal preference.

7. How much money do you want to spend and what terms can you set up? If you're the type of person who gets bored with an activity very soon after starting, it's wise to sign up for a short-term commitment, maybe even a trial plan. Don't lock yourself into an obligation that you don't want. See if you can join for three, six or nine months; you often can. It may cost a little more, but if you decide the club isn't for you, you save money in the long run.

8. If you think you may be moving before your contract expires, check the club's affiliations. Many clubs are part of a nationwide chain, which usually allows members to transfer their membership for a nominal charge, or even to use other facilities all over the nation — on a business trip or vacation, for instance. It's worth checking into.

9. Check the amenities available to you. Does the bathroom look as though it's well-stocked with everything that you will need? Many clubs offer the use of blow-dryers, curling irons and some even supply soap, shampoo, towels and sundry other items. The club may have listings of masseuses and other experts who might offer you a discount because of your membership in the club.

10. Is it close enough to your work or home so that you'll be able to get there with a minimum of hassles? Is there enough parking?

CREATE A HOME FITNESS CENTER

Maybe it's not practical for you to consider joining a health club. Your hours may be erratic, you may have a small child who requires that you be at home or, practically speaking, you may not be able to afford the prices being charged in your area. Not being able to join a health club is no excuse for not working out anymore. So pay attention; you may learn a few tricks here that will give you the motivation you need to get in shape in the comfort of your own home.

First, you need to find a suitable area in your home where you will be comfortable exercising. Think about what will be best for you; you may want privacy, you may want a nice view or you may prefer to find a place that's outside. Do whatever works for you; just make sure that the area that you pick is well-ventilated and that there's enough room for you to move about freely. You'll be running in place, jumping, dancing and flinging your arms.

Once you find the place, think about the way you want to decorate it. Since exercise and fitness are an important part of your life, you want to create an inviting atmosphere so that you can enjoy yourself while you're working out. Make your fitness fun! Try those inexpensive changes like painting the walls and adding brightly colored posters and inspirational photos. Hang a bulletin board where you can tack up key phrases and pictures that will help keep you motivated. Naturally, you'll want to hang a mirror (preferably full-length) and keep a tape measure handy so that your progress is noticed and recorded. Other amenities you'll want to consider include a floor mat or towel for floor exercises, and a ballet barre or a chair that you can put a leg on in order to fully stretch your leg muscles. Of course, a radio, tape player or record player will add some music while you work out. You may want to purchase some aerobic workout tapes for your fitness library so that you can vary your routine. There are many good ones sold with themes as varied as country-western, gospel and middle-of-the-road soft rock music.

Now that you've given some thought to the physical surroundings of your home fitness center, you should start to think how you'll want to equip it. The type of workout equipment you purchase depends on your interests, the exercises that work best for you and, again, the amount of money that you want to spend. You can get by with as little as a set of ankle weights and a jump rope, but other equipment to consider includes hand weights or barbells, a rebounder, a stationary bicycle, a broomstick or variations of these.

Hand weights. On the market you'll find weights especially made for women. They are shaped like a dumbbell and range from one to five pounds. If you're new to weight training, these might be just the thing for you. They are available at most sporting goods stores and many department stores, and are relatively inexpensive. Alternatives include canned goods of appropriate weights that you can hold in your hands, real dumbbells, or bleach bottles that have been filled with sand.

Barbells. Barbells are the time-honored tradition for weight training (also called free weights). They usually come in sets with the long bar and a couple of short bars for use as dumbbells. The flat weights that attach to the ends of the bars are called plates, and they range in weight from 2½ to twenty-five pounds. They are attached to the bar and held in place by collars.

Rebounder. The rebounder is relatively new on the market and isn't for everyone. It looks like a mini-trampoline and provides a springy surface for you to run in place comfortably. They are a great solution for people who are fairly out-of-shape, who don't feel comfortable about being seen running outdoors in shorts, so the rebounder offers privacy. The rebounder allows you to enjoy the benefits of running without the pounding and jarring of joints, commonly associated with running on hard surfaces. You can enjoy an aerobic dance routine — with all the jumps and kicks — on a rebounder for a change of pace. These usually retail for $75 to $150.

Stationary bicycle. There's nothing more convenient than being able to ride a stationary bicycle through a long, cold winter. You can maintain your aerobic fitness and muscle tone, easily and comfortably, and watch your friends turn to flab. My favorite workout routine on a stationary bike is to put on stereo headphones, turn on a favorite rock album and start cranking! It's easy to pedal for twenty to thirty minutes without even realizing how quickly time passes. Be sure to time yourself and record your progress from session to session. As you can imagine, working out on a stationary bike in a warm room can get you sweaty in a hurry, so keep a towel handy to mop up the perspiration as it trickles down your face. Dress appropriately, in either leotards or tights, and running or biking shoes. Or, if you'll feel more comfortable, wear biking shorts and a jersey for a real workout. Some people even like to catch up on their daily reading while on a bike.

An alternative to the stationary bicycle is rollers. They have been available for years to serious cyclists. Rollers require excellent cycling skills and a keen sense of balance; they're not suited for the novice cyclist.

Recently introduced on the market, however, is a training device that turns your bike into a stationary bike. Popular models are the Racer-Mate and TurboTrainer. These devices are bike stands on which you attach your road bike, minus the front wheel. They are sturdy, provide the required pedal resistance and are a good alternative to the traditional stationary bike. The benefit of rollers and bike stands is that you can become more used to your road bike, even though you're not out riding. When you get back on the streets you feel like you've been on your bike all winter long! Bike stands retail for about $150; a stationary bike can be bought for as little as $150, or for as much as $1000.

Broomstick. A broomstick or piece of dowel can prove valuable when performing certain exercises for your waist and stomach. Just grasp the stick in your hands, bring it over your head and stretch side to side. You can also put the stick on the floor and grasp it, working your hands up and down the shaft. This is great for the back and hamstrings.

Which Weights?

You may not know about all the different types of weight equipment on the market today. Basically, you have a choice between Nautilus, Universal and free weights. Each one offers certain benefits, and one or another may work out to be best for you. Why not give all three types of weights a try? You may even find that the best workout for you is a combination of all three systems. In any case, don't be intimidated by the array of impressive-looking machinery; ask questions and learn for yourself just how the machines work. It won't take long before you're a real pro at moving from one station to another, doing your repetitions, then moving on, just like you've been lifting weights all your life.

Two major rules to remember are:

1. Tone and trim — high repetitions, low weight.

2. Build and add bulk — high weight, low repetitions.

A series of weight-training exercises on Universal weight machines follows.

Cable Machine

The cable machine can help you strengthen and tone the muscles in the upper half of your legs. Although it may look confusing, the machine is easy to use. Just hook the leg strap cable onto the metal loop at the end of the cable and you're ready to attach it around your ankle. Buckle the leather strap so that it fits comfortably around your ankle, and you're ready to go.

Inner thighs. Stand up straight at arm's length from the machine with the strap fastened around your right ankle. Bring your right leg across the left foot; you should feel a pull in your inner thigh. Start this exercise with ten pounds of weight, and try to complete one set

Cable Machine: Inner Thighs

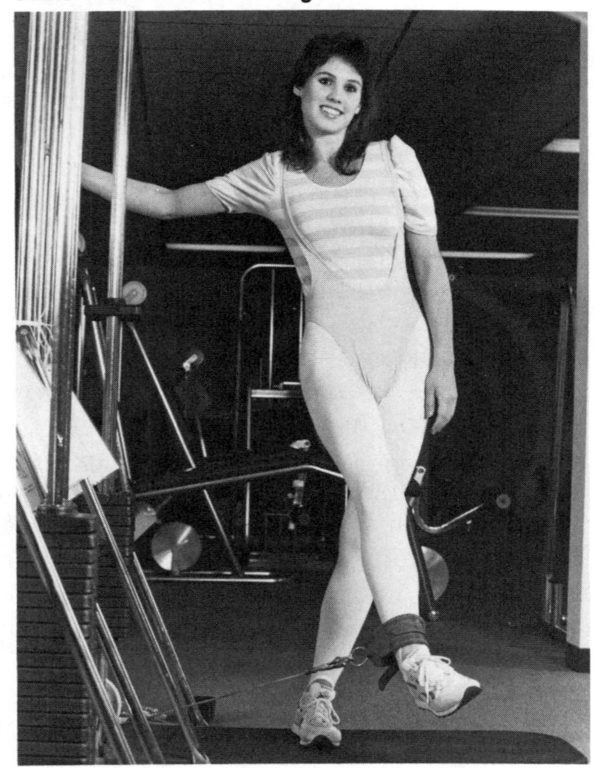

Use a light weight for working the inner thighs.

Cable Machine: Outer Thighs

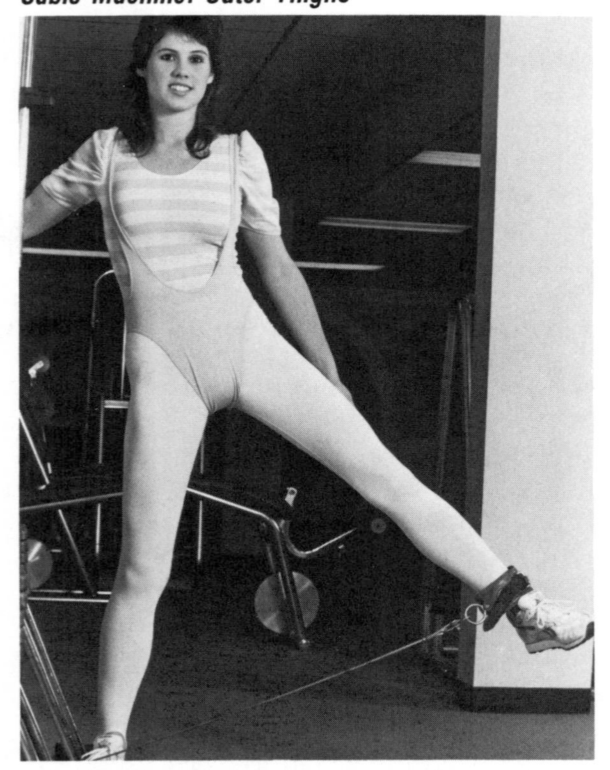

Working the outer thighs is a test of strength.

Cable Machine: Backs of Thighs

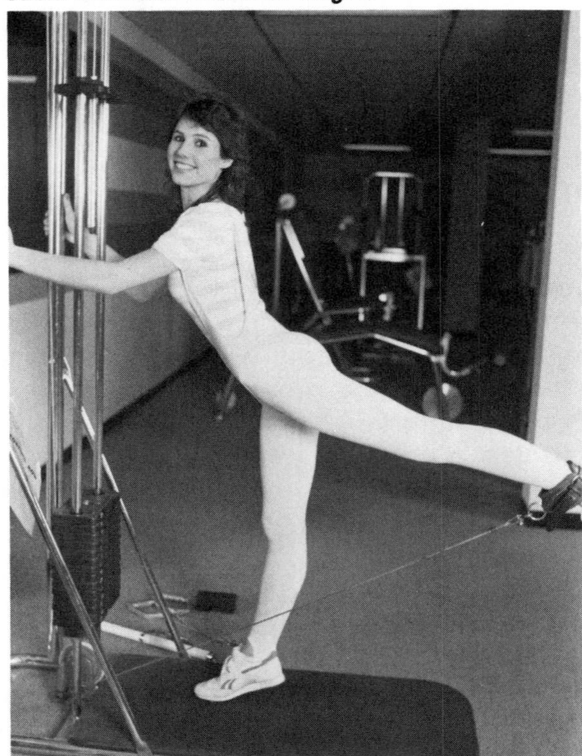

Don't drop the weight when you bring your leg down.

of twelve reps when you begin. This is one exercise where you can increase the number of sets that you do, but there's no need to increase the weight to more than ten pounds. Repeat the exercise with your left leg.

Outer thighs. Fasten the strap around your ankle once again, but this time you'll be moving your right leg away from your body, and feeling the movement in your upper/outer thigh. Again, you should have the weight at only ten pounds, and strive to increase the number of repetitions, not the amount of weight. Start with one set of twelve repetitions, and gradually increase the number of sets as you gain strength.

Back of the thigh. Fasten the strap comfortably around your right ankle and face the machine, holding onto the sides for balance. Bring your right leg back quickly; you only need to move it a few inches for this exercise to be effective. You'll feel it right away in the hamstrings. Do this exercise at ten pounds of weight, increasing the number of reps, not the amount of weight, as you become stronger.

Leg Press Machine: Quadriceps

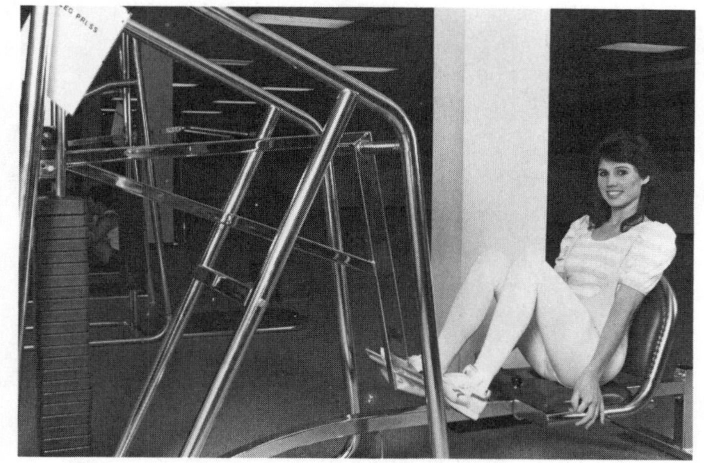

a. *The Leg Press Machine has an adjustable seat.*

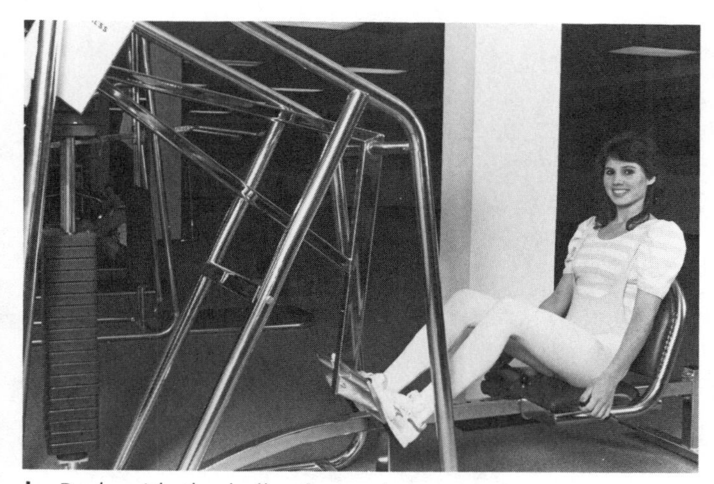

b. *Push with the balls of your feet.*

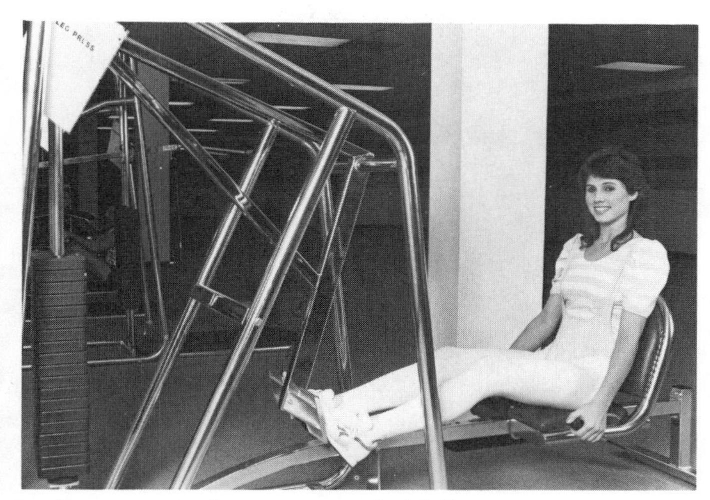

c. *Be sure your legs are extended fully.*

Leg Press Machine: Calves

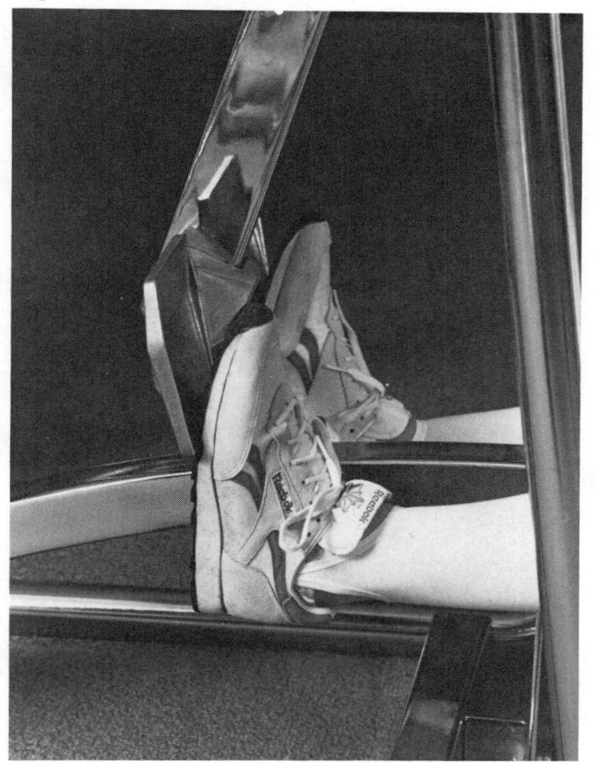

a. *To work the calves extend your legs.*

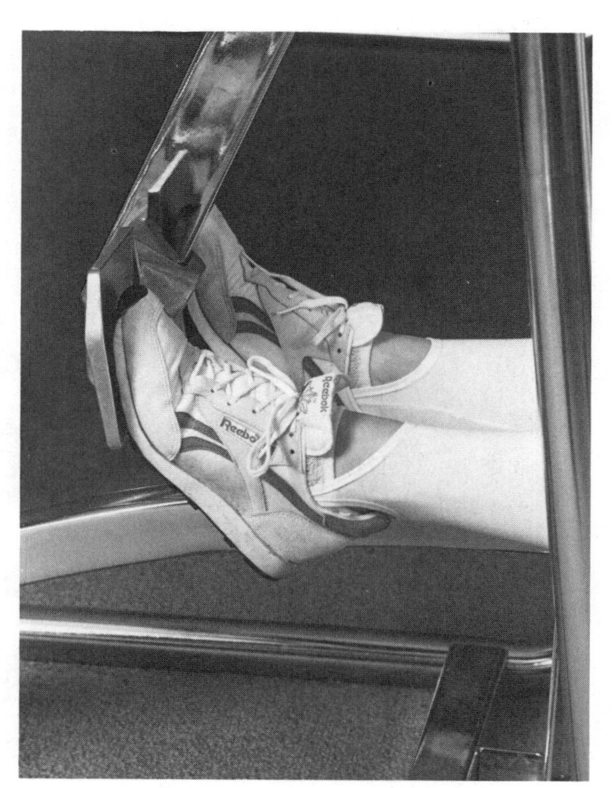

b. *Now flex your ankles back and forth.*

Leg Extension Machine: Quadriceps

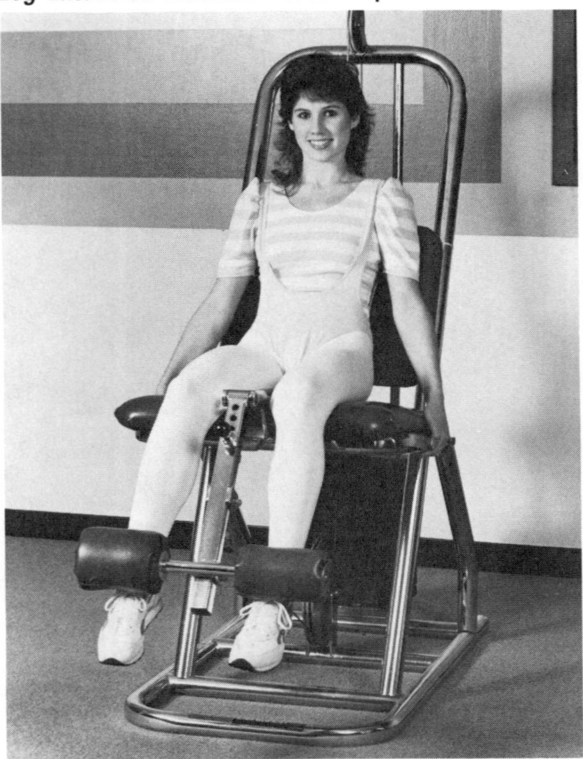

a. *The Leg Extension Machine has an adjustable setting for different leg lengths.*

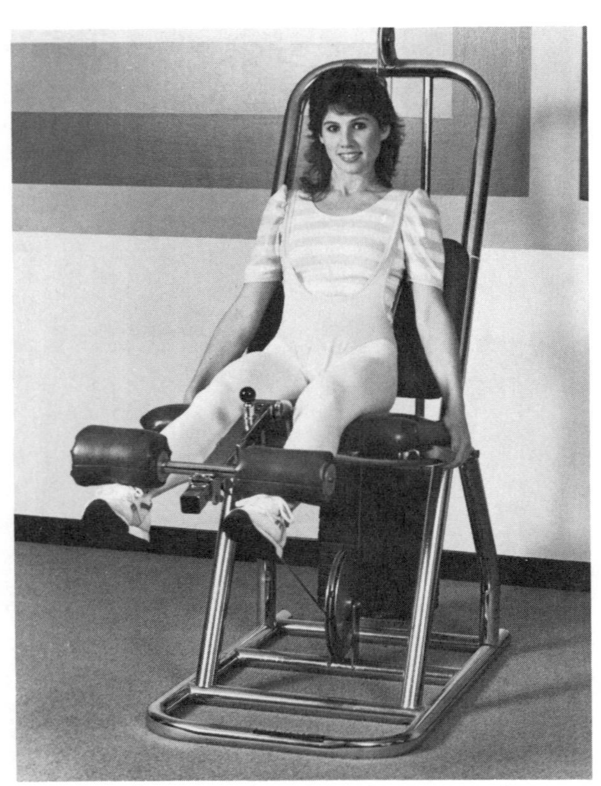

b. *Don't lift so much weight that you strain your knees.*

Leg Extension Machine: Hamstrings

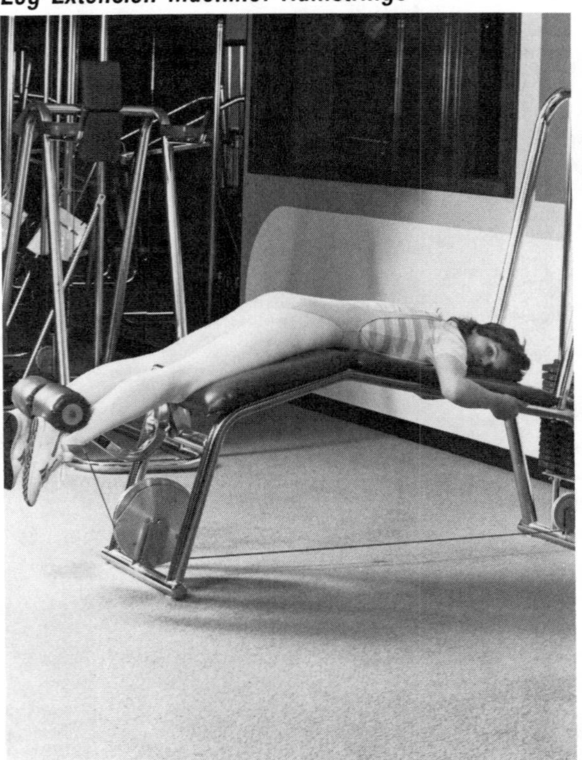

a. *Lie on your stomach when using the Leg Extension Machine.*

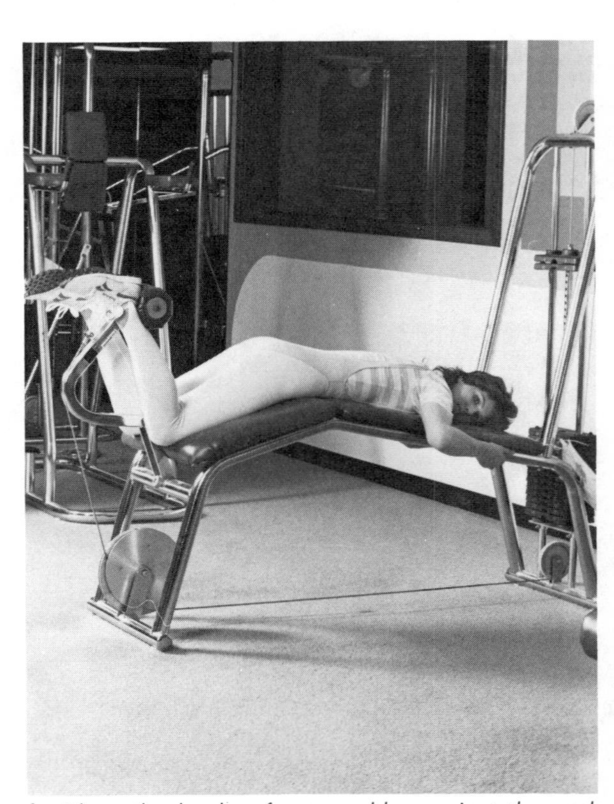

b. *Place the backs of your ankles against the pads and pull up.*

Leg Press Machine

The leg press machine will work on both your quadriceps and your hamstring muscles, as well as your calf muscles, depending on how you position your legs.

You can adjust the seat position for your body size. Pull the pin and move the chair either forward or backward, depending on what feels most comfortable for you. The pin slips right into the hole; it's very easy to reposition the seat. When you have the chair where you want it sit down and place your feet flat on the lower plates in front of you.

Quadriceps. It will take some trial and error at first to discover what weight is best for you, but start out with about forty to sixty pounds. This exercise is very simple; just push against the lower plates, exhaling as you press, inhaling as you release the weight carefully and gently. It's important to maintain control and to strive for smooth, easy movements. Start with one set of ten repetitions, increasing the amount of weight, number of reps and sets as your trainer advises.

Hamstrings. Position your feet this time on the upper plates, and again press as you did with the quadriceps exercise. You'll feel the exercise this time in the back of your thigh; start with one set of ten reps at the weight that feels comfortable.

Calf muscles. Position your feet on the lower plate and extend the legs at a comfortable weight. Instead of bringing them right back, for this exercise keep the legs extended and flex your feet against the plates, working the calf muscles. Start slowly with one set of ten reps, gradually increasing as it feels comfortable to you.

Leg Extension Machine

Another multi-purpose machine, the leg extension machine works both the quadriceps and the hamstrings. You'll notice two sets of padded bars — that's where you'll put your feet.

Quadriceps. Sit on the edge of the bench with your legs dangling, and feet placed securely under the lower padded bar. Lift the padded bar; your effort will come from the quadriceps. Extend your legs fully in front of you, then complete the exercise by bringing your legs back down. Do one set of twelve reps, increasing the number of sets and repetitions as you feel stronger. It is easy to bulk up here, so don't use a lot of weight.

Hamstrings. Lie face down on the bench with your legs straight back behind you, feet positioned under the padded bar. Bring your legs back toward your body and then return to the original position for one repetition. This exercise strengthens and tones the entire back of the thigh — a problem spot for many women. Again, it's important to start slowly, both with the number of repetitions and the amount of weight that you use.

8 LEG AND THIGH EXERCISES

All the Leg Lifts and Donkey Kicks in the world won't burn fat just from your thighs. But the spot exercises that you perform for your legs, thighs, calves and ankles do have a beneficial effect on the size and shape of your body. However, remember to think of your body in terms of a whole, not a series of little trouble spots that can be whittled away.

Spot exercises, because they burn energy, are good for your entire body. Remember, any movement that gets your heart pumping is great for you. And, because the spot exercise is designed to work specific parts of your legs, it does strengthen and tone the muscles. So taking a floor exercise class, participating in aerobic exercise or just working out on your living room floor for an hour every day will help tone, trim and improve the appearance and fitness of your legs and thighs.

It is important to do the exercises correctly in order to get the most out of them. You don't want to exhaust yourself, but you should work hard enough so that you can see some results. You may feel a burning sensation in your muscles when you work them very hard. The burning sensation comes from a buildup of lactic acid, a waste product of exercise in the muscles. The muscles hurt when the body can't remove the lactic acid as fast as it is produced. The burning will subside quickly, if you take a few deep breaths, stretch the sore area for a moment and then continue with your routine. Oxygen helps carry the waste products away from the muscles.

Pay attention to your posture while you do the exercises; also, be sure to keep your hands under the small of your back when you're lying on your back. Too many women do not take care of their lower backs, and end up injuring themselves. Always support your lower back.

When you do the exercises, always dress in clothing that does not restrict movement. Have a towel handy and, if you're exercising on a bare floor, you might want to invest in an exercise mat or large beach towel for added cushioning and warmth.

Turn on some music to help you with your routine. There's nothing like a rock and roll tune to help rev you up and keep you going. Some suggested albums are:

PERFORMER	ALBUM NAME	LABEL
Michael Jackson	"Off the Wall"	Epic Records
Olivia Newton-John	"Physical"	MCA Records
Diana Ross	"Why do Fools Fall in Love?"	RCA Records
Stray Cats	"Built for Speed"	EMI America
The Cars	"The Cars"	Elektra
Tubes	"The Completion Backward Principle"	EMI Records
Bruce Springsteen	"The River"; "Darkness on the Edge of Town"	Columbia Records

For slower, sustained stretches:

Barry DeVorzon and Perry Botkin, Jr.	"Nadia's Theme"	A & M Records
Boz Skaggs	"Silk Degrees"	Columbia Records
Luther Vandross	"Never Too Much"	Epic Records
John Klemmer	"Touch"	MCA Records
James Galway	"Songs of the Seashore"	RCA Records

Remember that when you're stretching, you should try to maintain a smooth movement. Do not bounce! If you bounce while you are stretching, you can easily injure yourself. This is called a ballistic movement. Stretching should be a *slow, sustained* movement. Stretching before and after your regular routine will help you to lengthen those muscles that you work so hard; it also helps to prevent cramping and soreness by loosening your muscles.

So pick and choose the exercises that best suit you. And remember that you can exercise at any time of day. For instance, while you're brushing your teeth, it's very easy to do a few calf raises. Learn to use your time creatively in similar ways. What else can you be doing when you automatically incorporate exercise into your routine? You can do Knee Bends while washing the dishes, you can dance while you're on the phone, you can do Wall Bends while waiting for a friend. Give it some thought and you'll be amazed by how many opportunities you'll have to really move through your days!

What follows is a series of leg exercises that will get your blood flowing and slim you down. Pick and choose a couple from each category to create a routine that is both fun and effective.

General Exercises

Jumping Jacks. Stand tall, feet together, hands at sides. Simultaneously spring up, spreading your legs. Coordinating that motion, bring your hands over your head, arms straight. Now bounce again, bringing legs and arms back to the starting position. Keep your legs straight throughout the motion. This is a good warmup. Do twenty.

(2 photos)

Squat Thrusts. From a standing position, quickly squat, bending at the knees. Then thrust your legs out and straight behind you; return to a squatting position by thrusting your legs back. Do fifteen. To make this one more difficult, when your legs are straight behind you, spread them in one bouncing motion, then back in; continue as before.

(2 photos)

Aerobic Action. The number of fun jumping exercises that you can do to music is limitless. Try jumping in place or skipping in place. Touch your elbow to your opposite knee as you dance/jump to your favorite tunes. Practice your footwork; try some fancy moves like shuffle steps across the room. Any exercise that gets your heart pumping, lets you sweat just a bit and uses your muscles will be doing you some good. So be creative and make up your routine as you go along — have fun!

Jumping Jacks

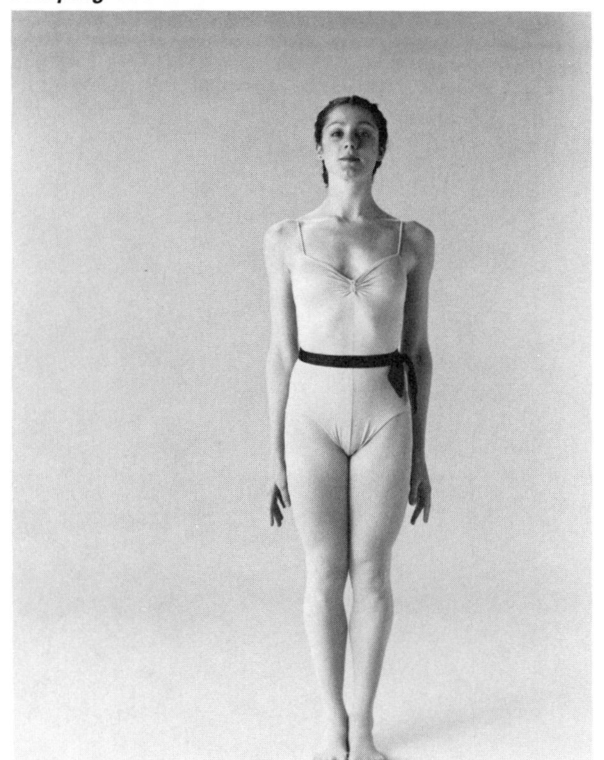

a. *Begin Jumping Jacks with hands at sides.*

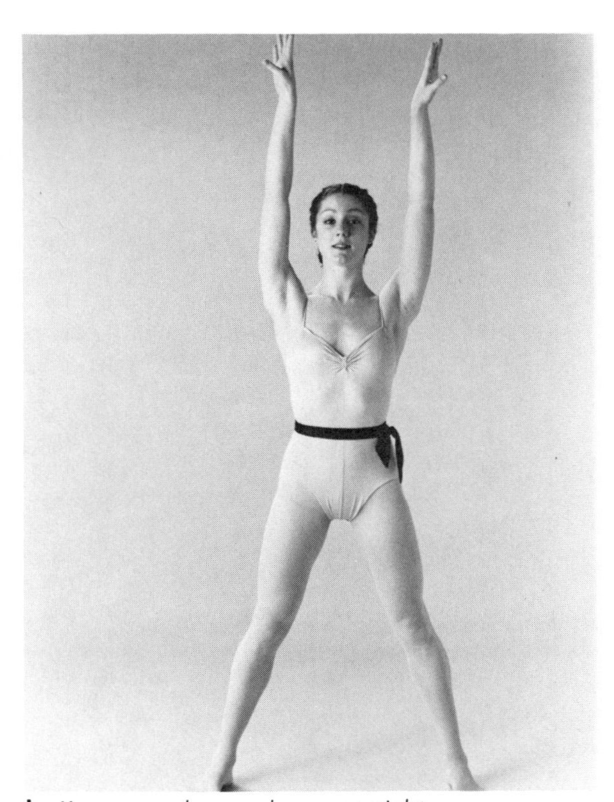

b. *Keep your legs and arms straight.*

Squat Thrusts

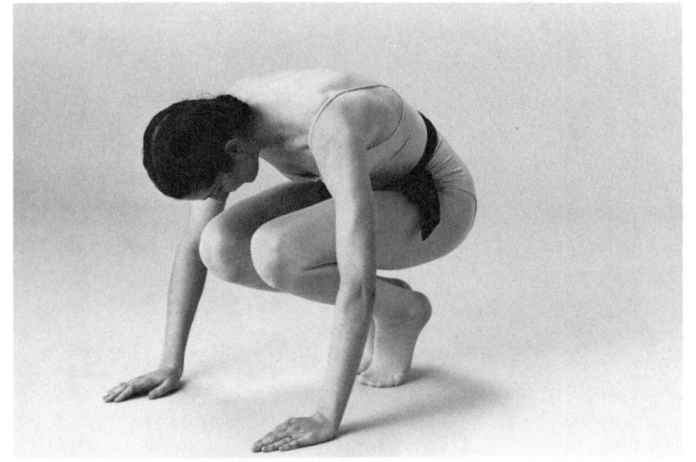

a. *Squat Thrusts build the arms as well as the legs.*

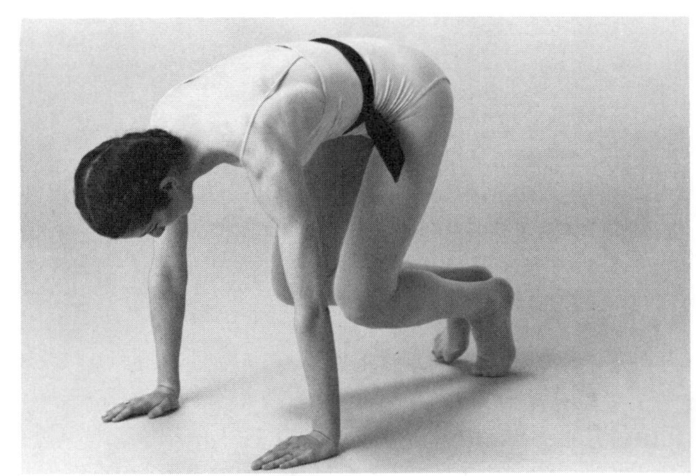

b. *Be sure to extend your legs fully.*

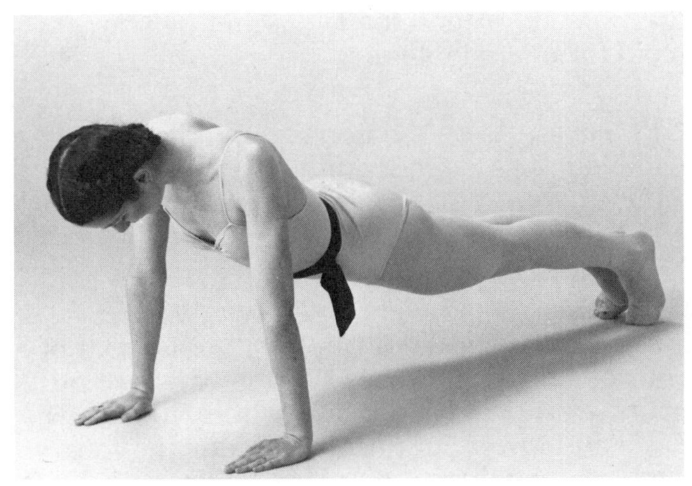

c. *For variety, spread your legs when they're extended.*

Aerobic Action

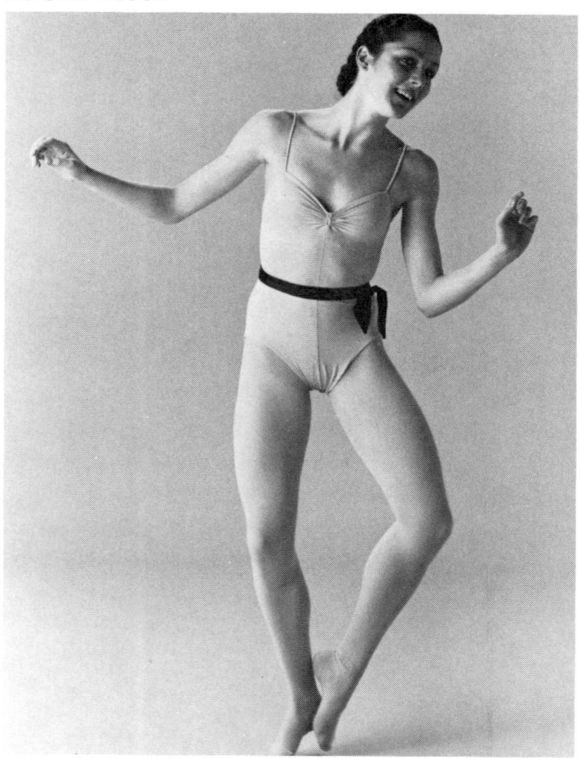

Any activity that increases your heart rate is good for you.

Calf Muscles

Calf Stretch. Lean against a wall with your palms flat, extending your feet behind you, keeping them flat on the floor. Extend your right leg behind you. Feel the stretch, return the leg, then repeat with the left leg. To intensify the stretch, move your hands farther down the wall and extend the leg farther behind you. Hold for one minute.

Calf Flexes. Sit on the floor or on a hard chair with your legs extended in front of you. Point and flex your feet, keeping your legs straight and tight. Do five.

Calf Raises. Stand with legs about two feet apart. Place your hands on the floor in front of you, bending your knees slightly. Now extend your hands on the floor, away from your body. Raise and lower your heels, working the muscles in your calves and ankles. Do five.

Calf Flexes

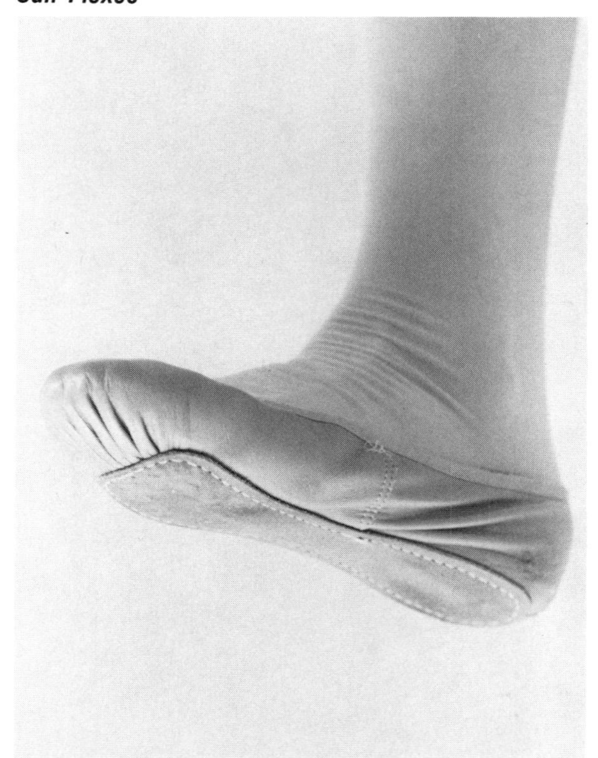

a. *Flex the ankle to flex the calf muscles.*

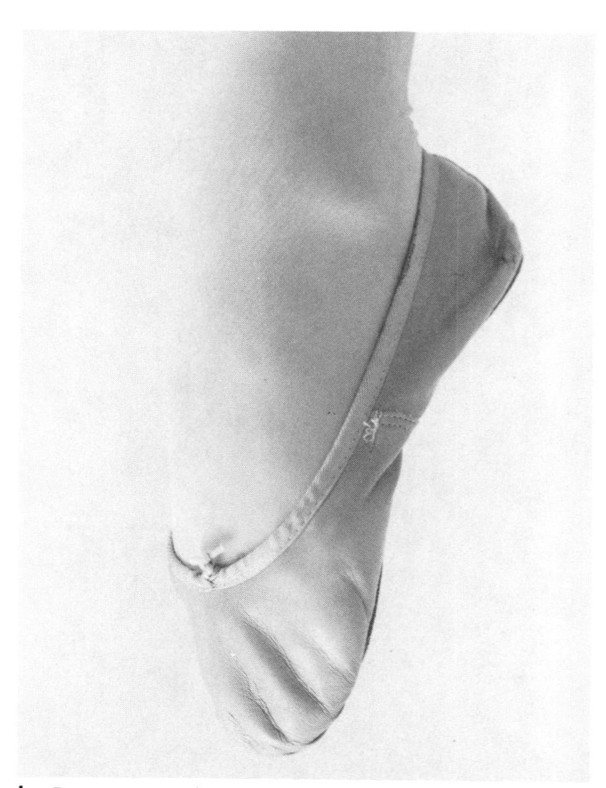

b. *Be sure you have a full range of motion.*

Calf Raises

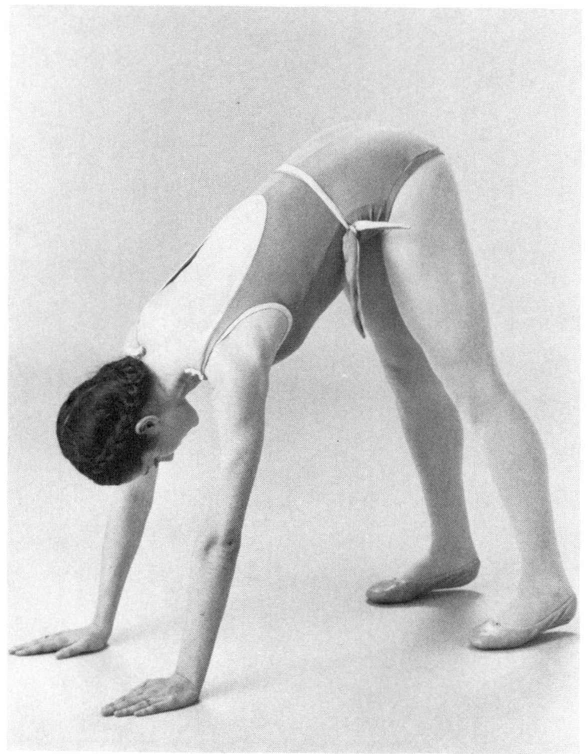

a. *Begin Calf Raises with hands and feet on the floor.*

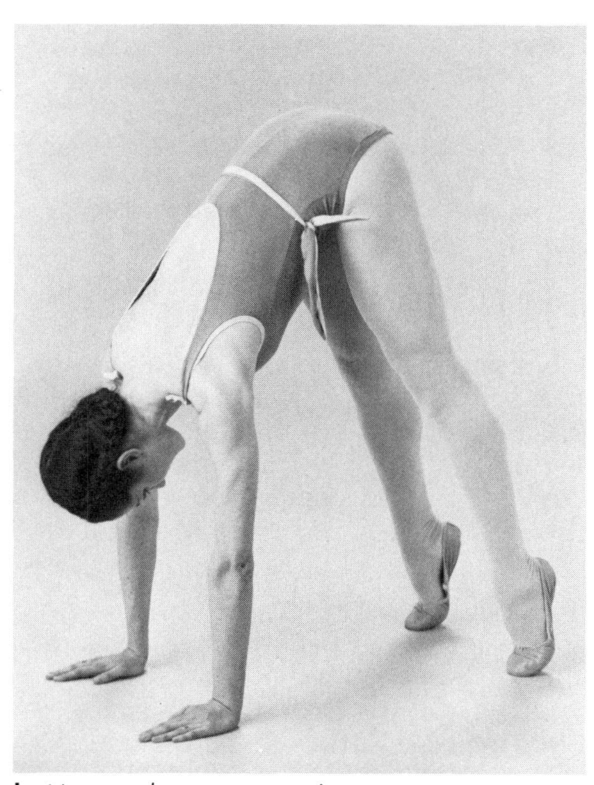

b. *Now push up on your tiptoes.*

Inner Thigh Stretch

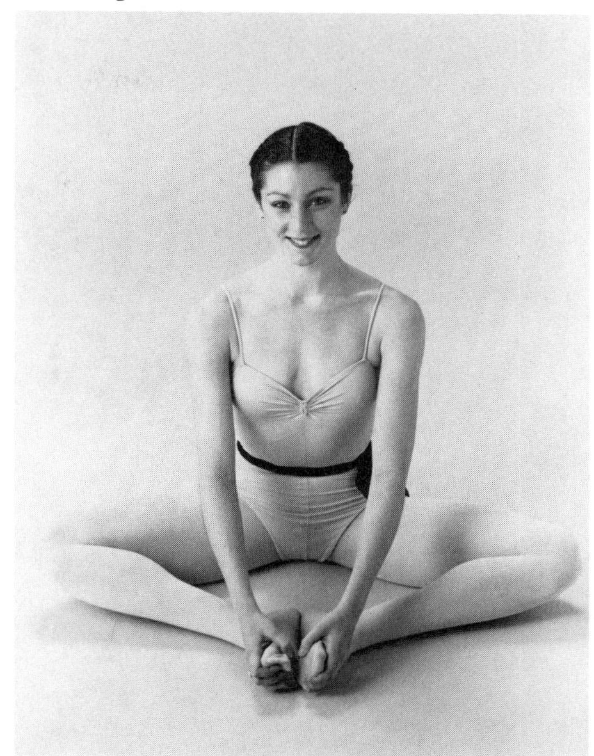

This is the ultimate pose for Inner Thigh Stretch. But don't overdo it.

Inner Thighs

Inner Thigh Stretch. Sit up straight on the floor and bring the soles of your feet together. Gently bring your feet as close to your groin area as possible, bending at the knees. Place your elbows on your knees and try to push your knees to the floor. Feel the pull in your inner thigh. Gently ease off, then push again. Do for one minute.

Butterflies. Assume the same position as above, but *gently* move your legs up and down as you continue to stretch the inner thigh. This exercise will help increase flexibility in your inner thighs and also to tone and stretch the muscles.

Leans. Spread your legs in front of you on the floor while sitting up straight; spread them as far apart as you can, then lean forward from the waist. Stretch your hands out in front of you, then place one hand on each foot; stretch again from the waist. Hold for thirty seconds.

Butterflies

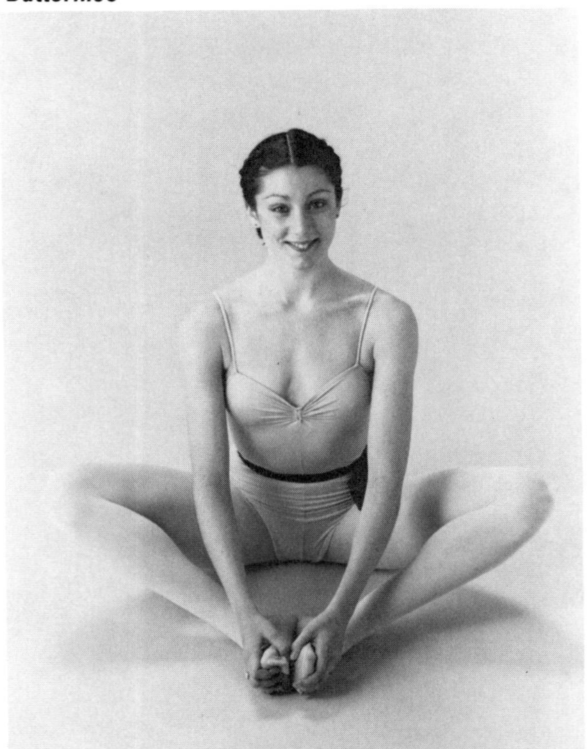

a. *Butterflies are active Inner Thigh Stretches.*

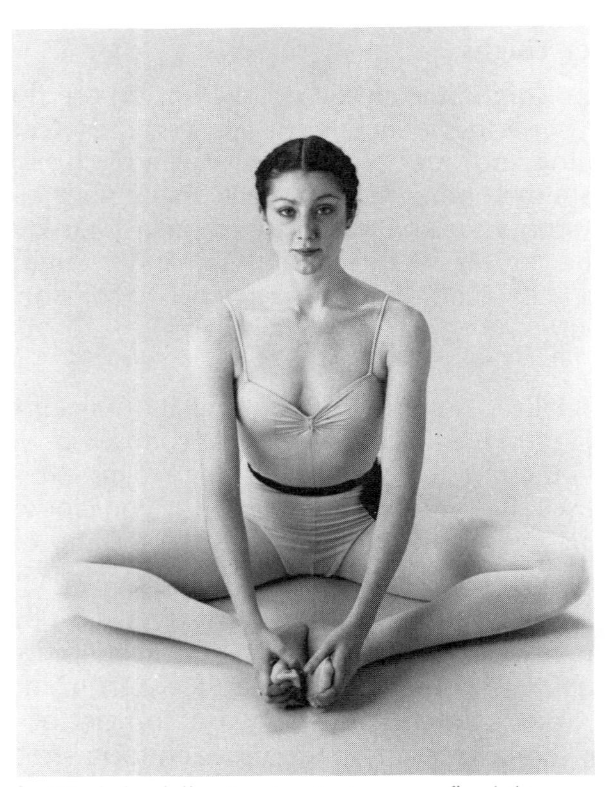

b. *Work for full extension to increase flexibility.*

Leans

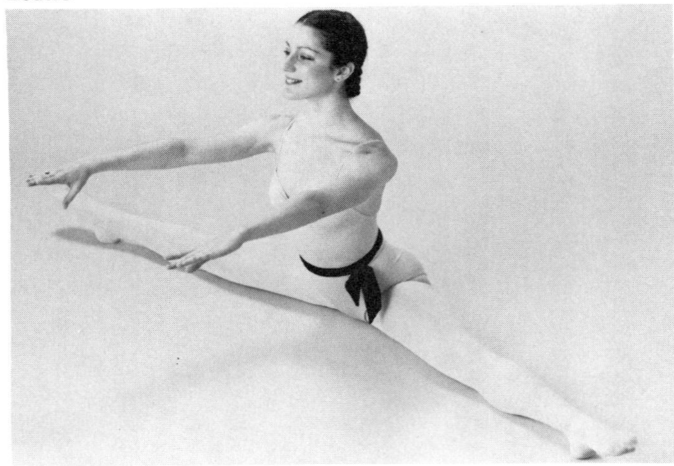

a. *Spread your legs wide for Leans.*

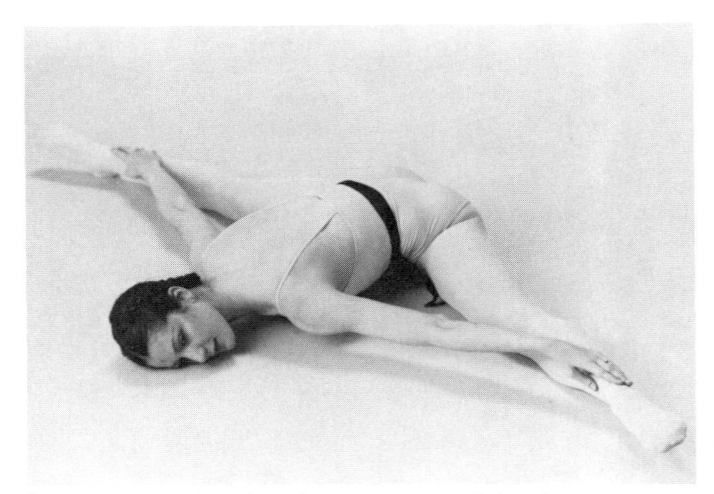

b. *Now try to bend at the waist toward the floor.*

Killer Inner Thigh Lifts. Lie on your right side on the floor, both legs extended, side by side. Now bring the left leg over the right, placing the foot flat on the floor with your leg bent at the knee. Point the right foot and raise the entire leg up and down in small movements. Be sure to keep the leg straight. Do ten with the foot pointed, then flexed. Switch sides and repeat the series with the left leg.
(2 photos)

Scissors. Lie on your back with your hands under the small of your back. Bring your legs up perpendicular to the floor, then separate them, with feet flexed. Quickly criss-cross your feet four times, then separate your legs into a "V"; quickly bring them back, and criss-cross again. Do five with your feet flexed, then repeat with the toes pointed.

Killer Inner Thigh Lifts

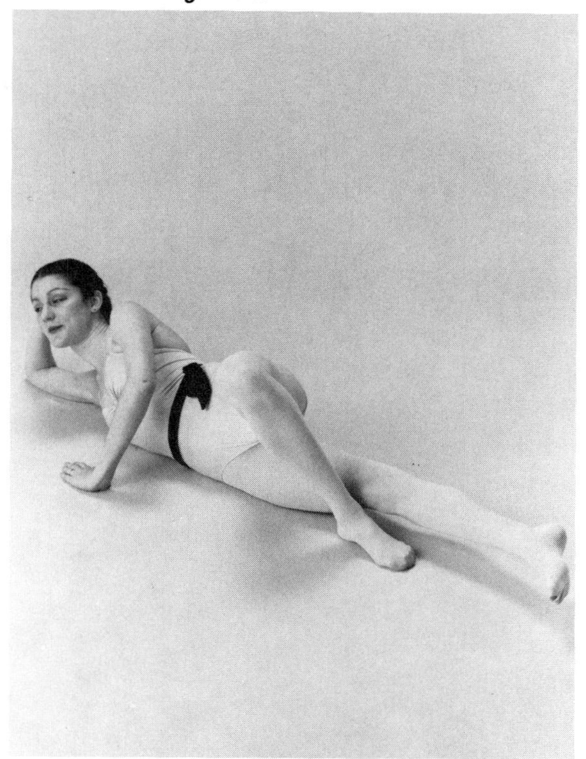

a. *Killer Inner Thigh Lifts are a real challenge.*

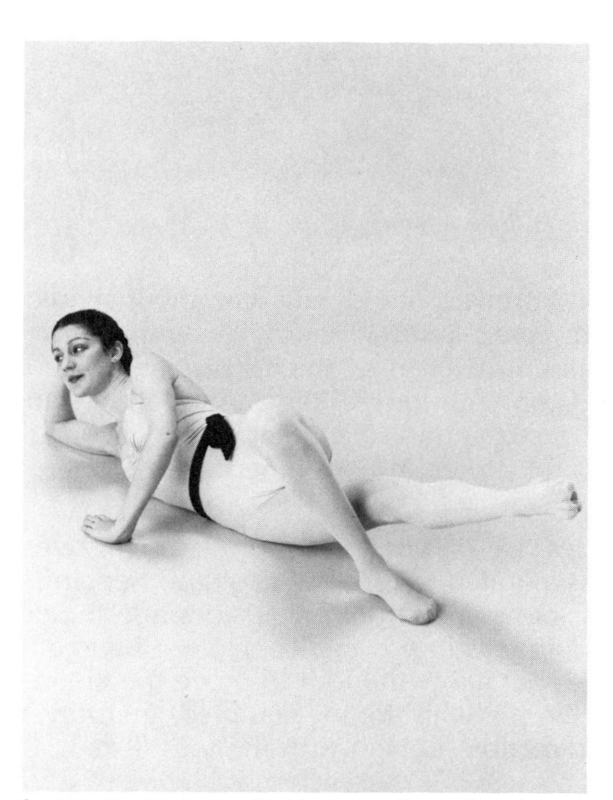

b. *Lift the leg just a few inches off the floor.*

Scissors

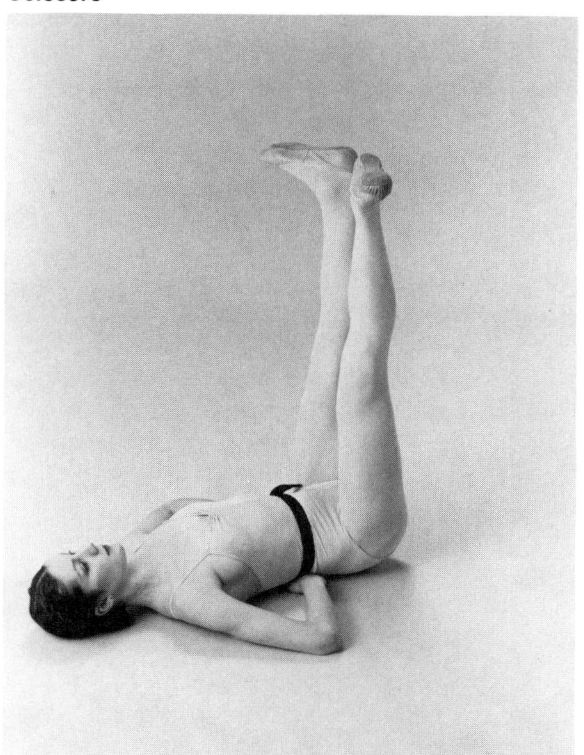

a. *When doing Scissors, keep your hands behind your back.*

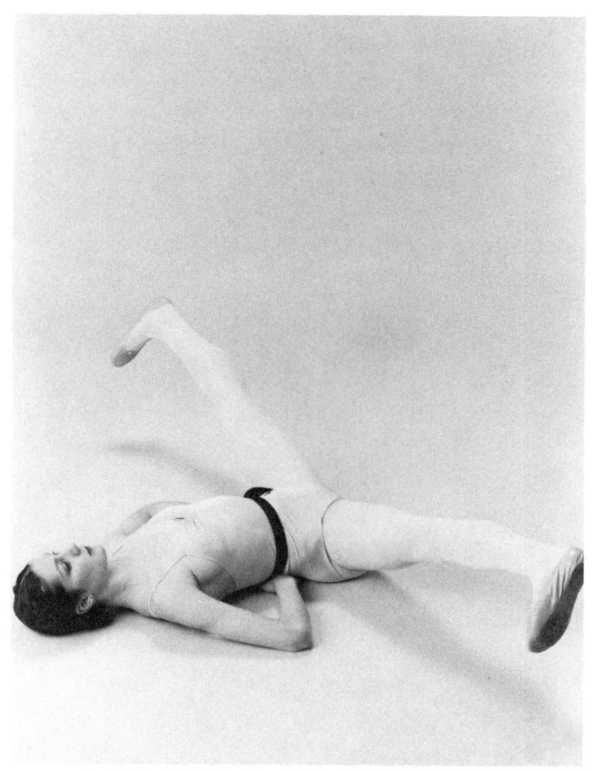

b. *Spread your legs as wide as you can.*

Little Bounces

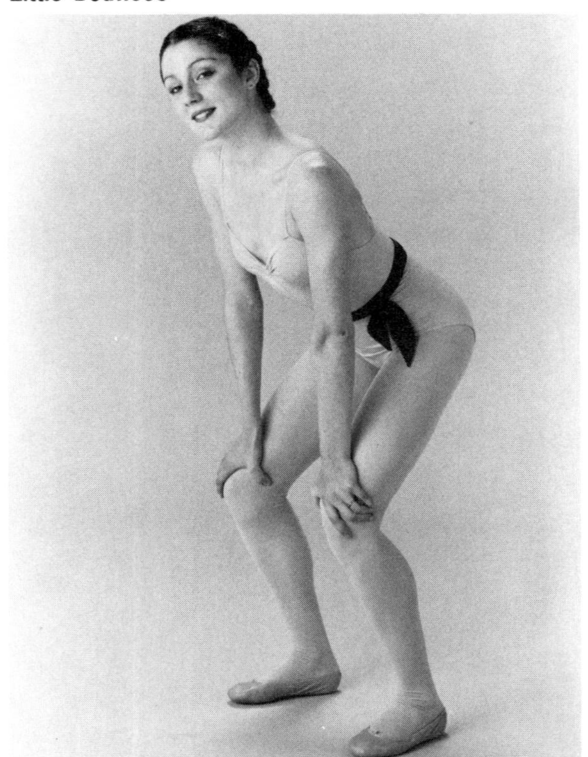

Don't strain your knees doing Little Bounces.

Circles

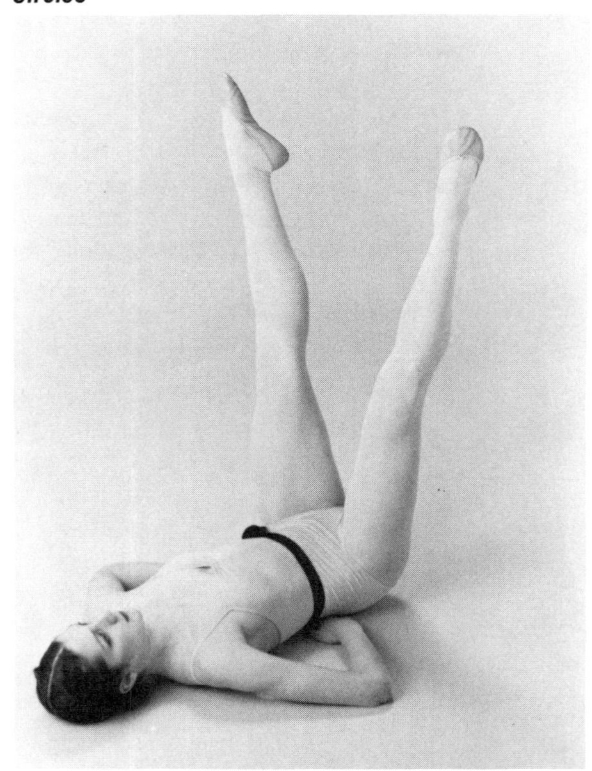

Assume the position of Scissors to do Circles.

Inner Thigh Leg Lift

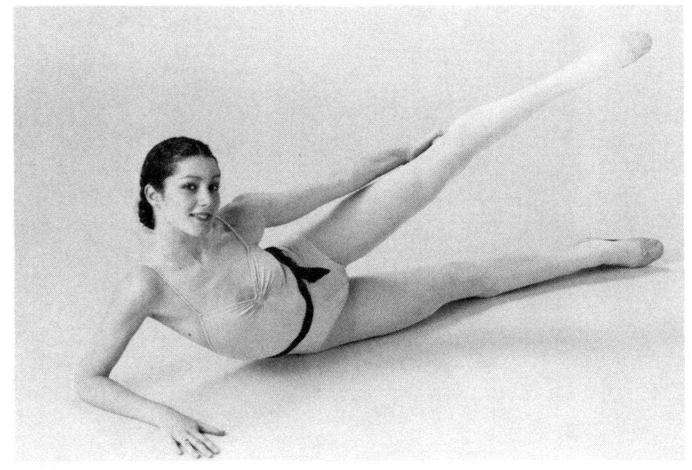

a. *First bring one leg up.*

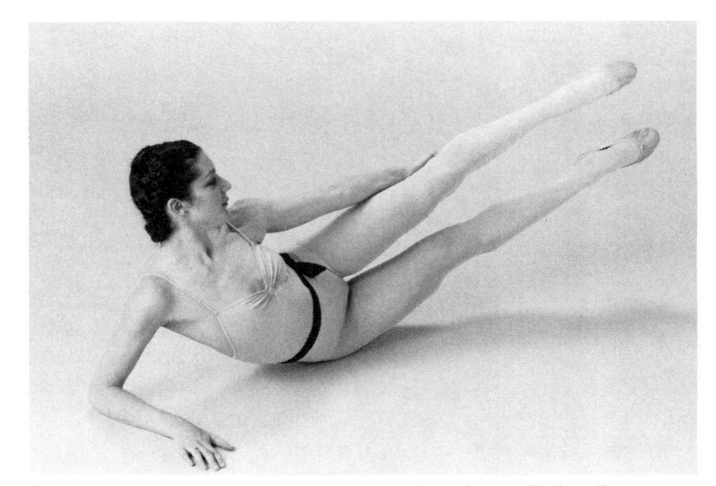

b. *Now bring the other leg several inches off the floor.*

Little Bounces. Stand with feet about shoulder-width apart. Bend at your knees until you feel the pull in your inner thighs, placing your hands on your knees. Repeat motion of standing up straight and bending, gently, feeling the pull and stretch in your inner thigh. Do ten.

Circles. Lie on your back with legs elevated and separated in the "V" position. Keeping your legs straight, point your toes and move the feet and legs in tiny circles. Do not bend at the ankle, but allow the foot to move the entire leg. Do ten with the toes pointed, then reverse the direction. Repeat with the toes flexed.

Inner Thigh Leg Lift. Lie on right side, lift your left leg up and keep it straight. Prop yourself up with your right hand and elbow on the floor.

Side Leg Lunges

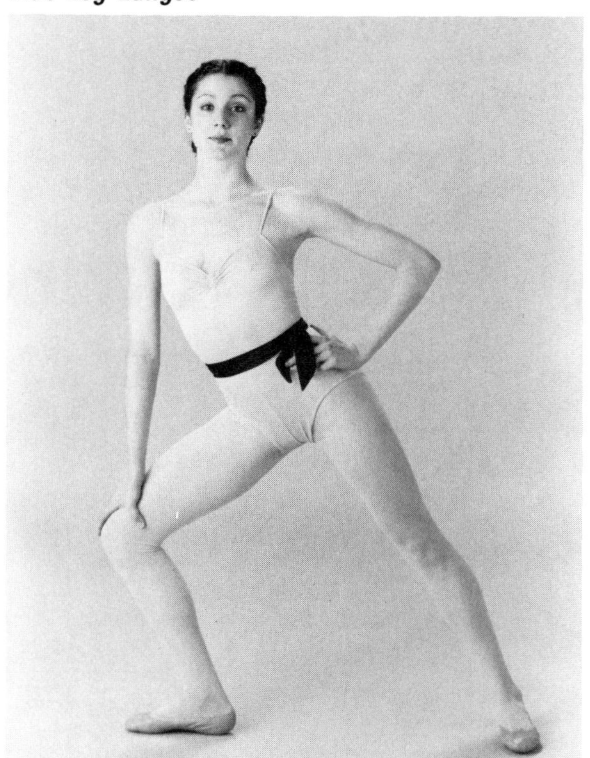

Side Leg Lunges are used in yoga.

Hold your leg at your knee with your right hand, if you need to. Bring your right leg up to meet your left, moving it smoothly and strongly. Return your legs to the floor. Repeat. Try to do thirty. Repeat, turning onto your left side, bringing your left leg up to meet your right leg.

Side Leg Lunges. Stand straight and spread your legs about three feet apart. Now turn one foot so that it forms a right angle with the other. Bend at the knee the leg with the foot you just turned to make a right angle. Now put the hand nearest the bent leg on the knee. Then stretch your other straight leg. Use the bent leg for support. Hold for a count of ten. Return to an upright position and repeat to the right ten times. Then do the left leg. This exercise stretches the inner thigh and strengthens the opposite quadriceps.

Back of the Thigh

Donkey Kicks. There are a number of variations to this exercise; it is one of the most effective exercises that you can do for toning your thighs. On hands and knees, bring your right knee to your nose, then extend your leg back,

Donkey Kicks

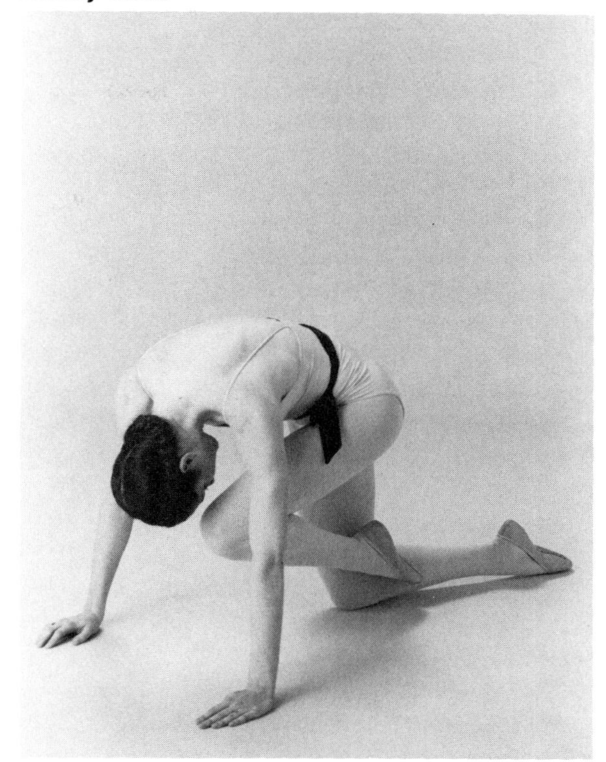

a. *Start in this position for Donkey Kicks.*

stretching it as far as you can; keep it straight and tight. Do twenty-five, then do twenty-five with the left leg.

On hands and knees, stretch your right leg back as far as you can, keeping it straight. Then lift the leg from the buttock without bending the knee. Don't worry about getting the leg up very far; just do little kicks, about ten. Repeat with the left leg.

On hands and knees, extend your right leg back behind you. This time, though, instead of extending the leg straight back, bend it at the knee, pointing the toes toward the ceiling. Lift the leg up from the hip; you don't need to move very far to get good results. Do fifteen, then repeat with the left leg. Repeat with the foot flexed.

A good stretch to try after Donkey Kicks: Tuck your legs, knees bent and sitting upright. Stretch s-l-o-w-l-y from one side to the other by leaning, feeling the stretch in your upper thigh, where it probably hurts the most. Hold for one minute.

Donkey Kick, Cont'd.

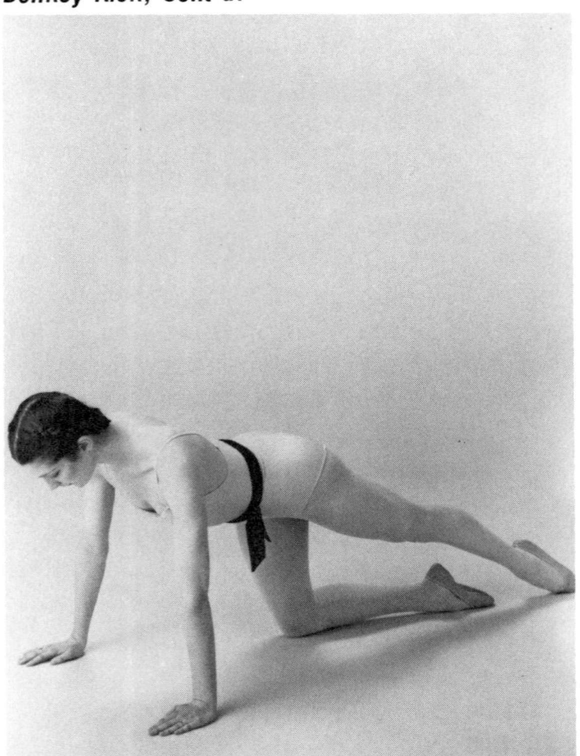

b. *Extend the leg behind you.*

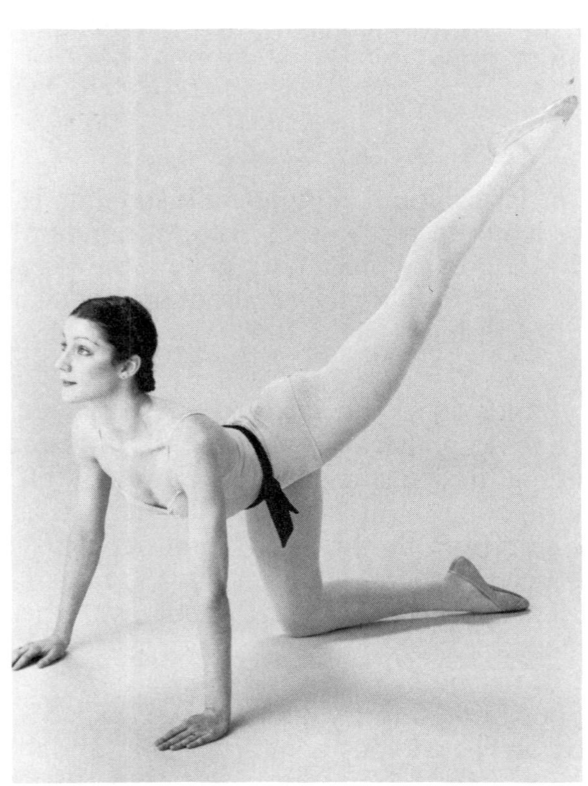

c. *Now raise the leg.*

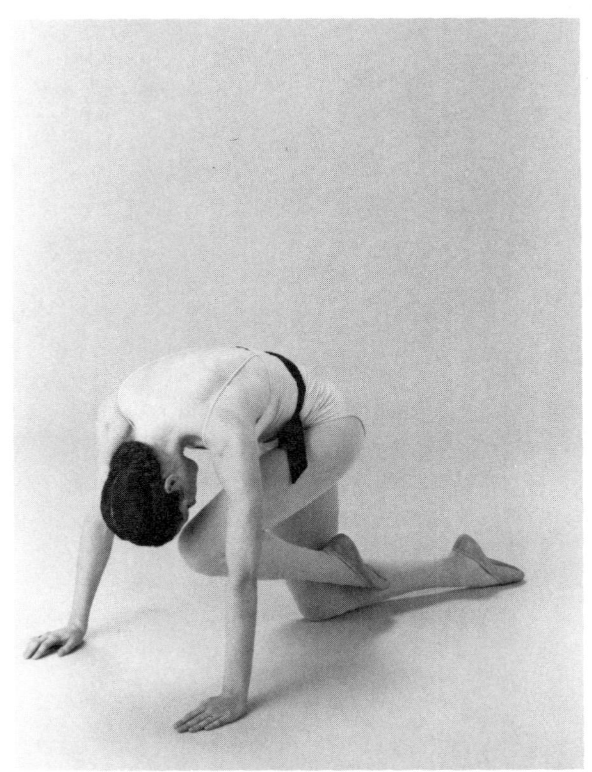

d. *Return to your starting position.*

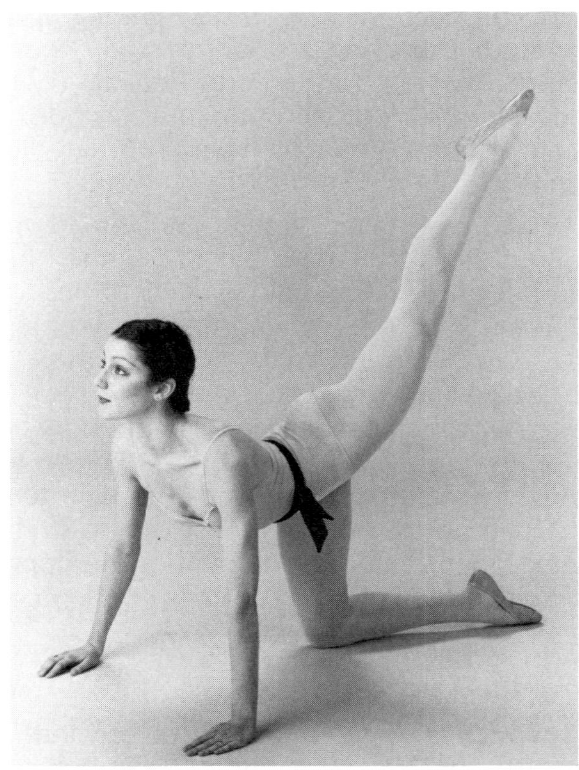

e. *In this variation, begin with the leg extended and move it up and down.*

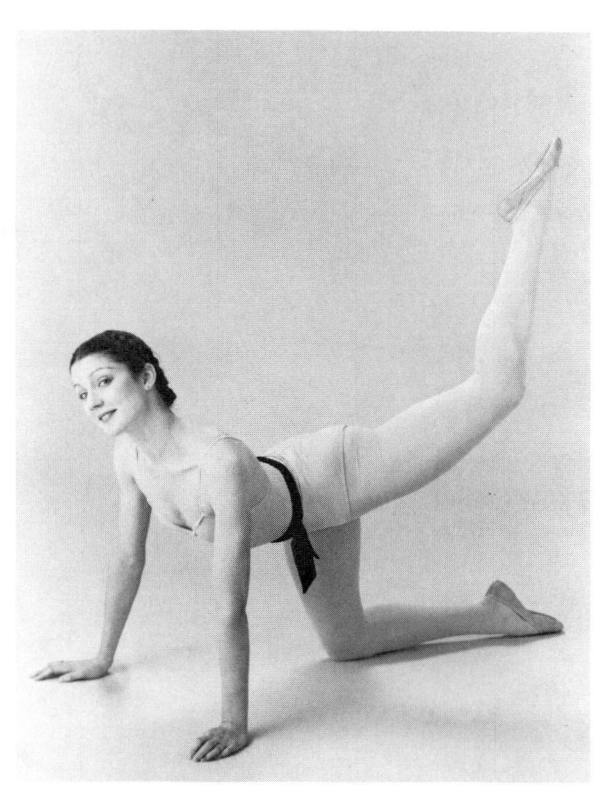

f. *Keep your knee bent and move the leg up and down.*

Hamstring Stretch

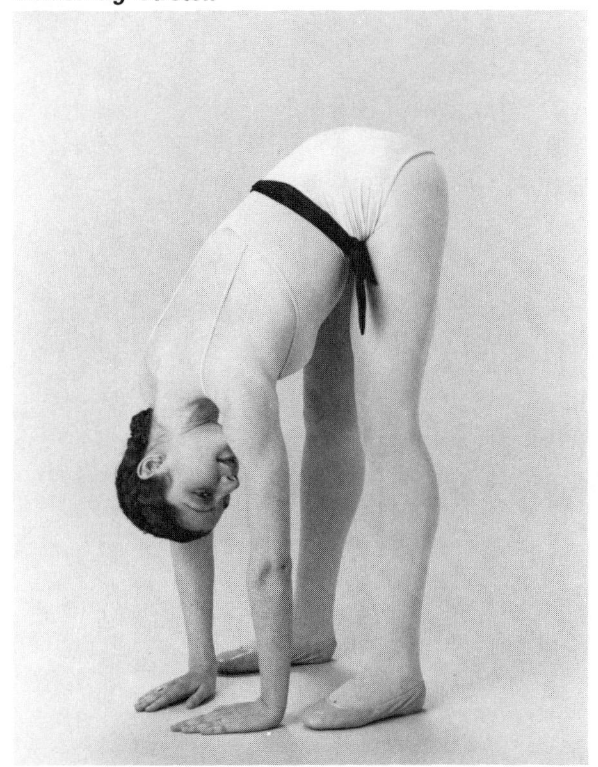

If you can keep this pose in the Hamstring Stretch, you're very flexible.

Hamstring Stretch. With both feet flat on the floor, reach down and try to touch your toes. Then, separate your feet and put your palms on the floor. Move smoothly — no jerking or bouncing allowed. Feel the pull in the back of your thighs — it will help to lengthen and stretch those muscles. Hold for one minute.

Up and Back. With your feet about shoulder-width apart, bend your knees and swing your arms through your legs, then go back to a standing position. Repeat. Do fifteen to build endurance and strength in your hamstrings. This one also helps build endurance in the quadriceps.

Floor Lunge. Place your hands on the floor and extend your legs behind you; put your weight on your hands and toes, keeping your body straight. Bring the right leg forward, even with your right hand with the right knee bent, left leg extended back. Feel the stretch in your legs — hold the position for thirty seconds, then repeat the movement with your left leg. When you've stretched both legs, shift position so that both hands and feet are flat on the floor; bring the right leg forward, with your foot near your right hand, keep both legs straight, stretch, then repeat the movement with the left leg forward.

Double V. Start out with both hands and feet on the ground about shoulder-width apart, keeping your legs straight. Slowly walk the legs toward the hands, feeling the stretch in the back of your legs. Be sure to keep your legs straight. Do for one minute.

Pretzel Toe Touch. To get a good stretch in your hamstrings, cross your legs at the knees and then touch your toes. Feel the stretch and gently push just a little farther. Hold for thirty seconds.

Backward Toe Touches. Start off with your knees bent and your hands on the floor; then gently straighten your legs, keeping your hands on the floor. Do ten.

Up and Back

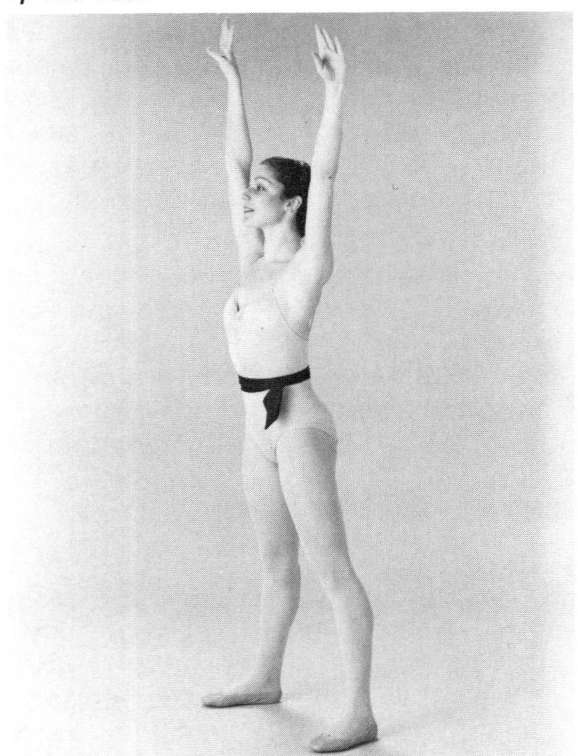

a. *Up and Back is great for increasing flexibility.*

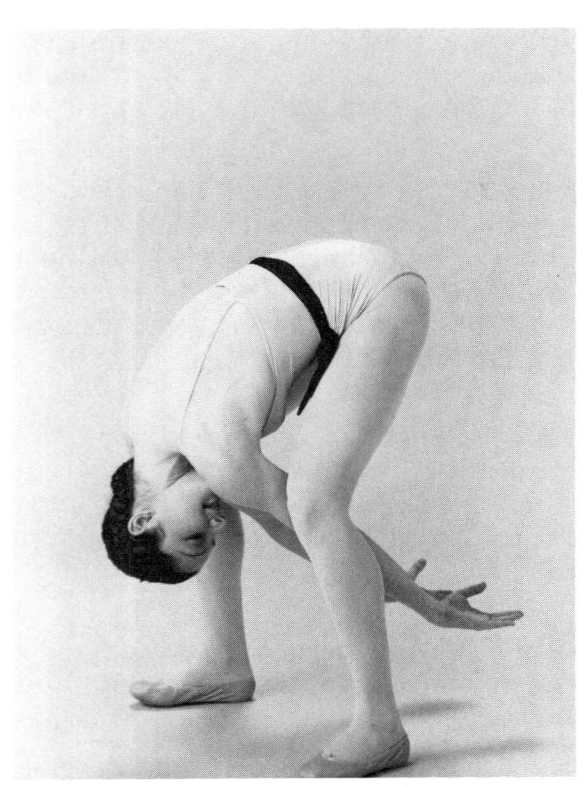

b. *Bring your arms down and back as far as you can.*

Floor Lunges

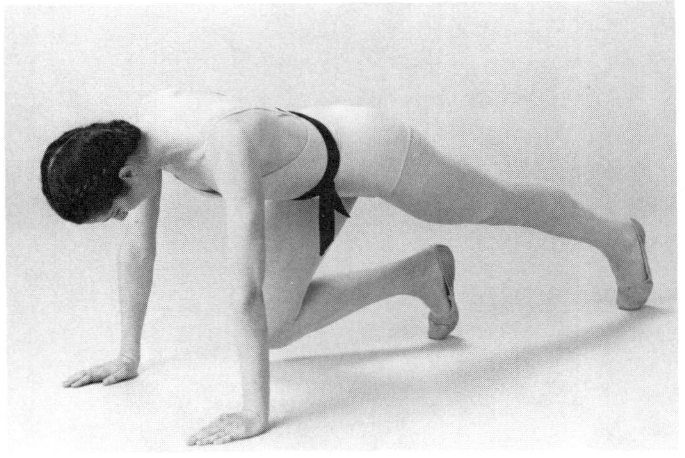

a. *The start of a Floor Lunge is like a sprinter's pose.*

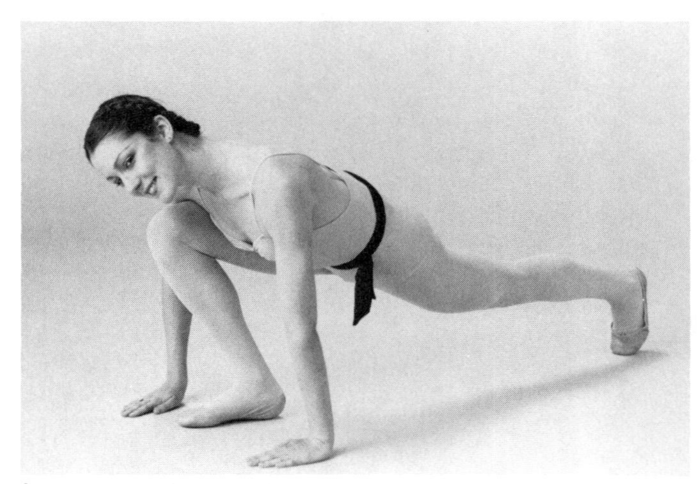

b. *You can alternate legs.*

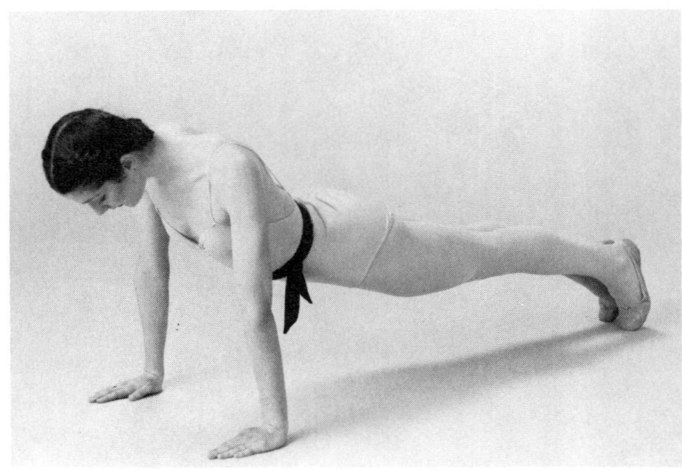

c. *Be sure both legs are extended before starting the next lunge.*

Double V

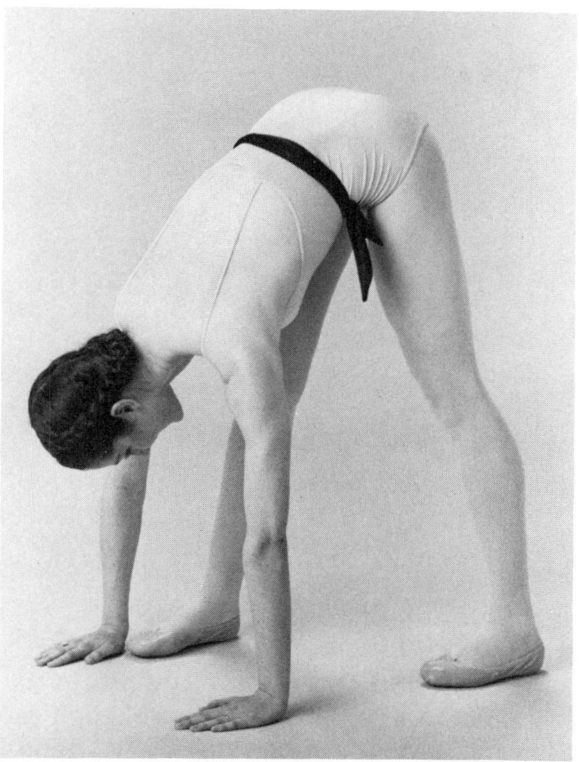

Begin the Double V with your legs far from your hands; bring your feet forward without bending the knees.

Pretzel Toe Touches

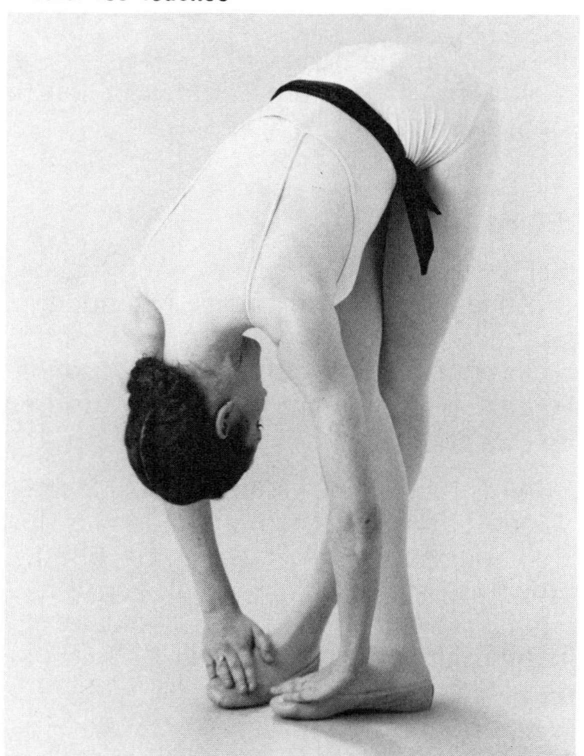

Alternate leg positions when doing the Pretzel Toe Touch.

Backward Toe Touches

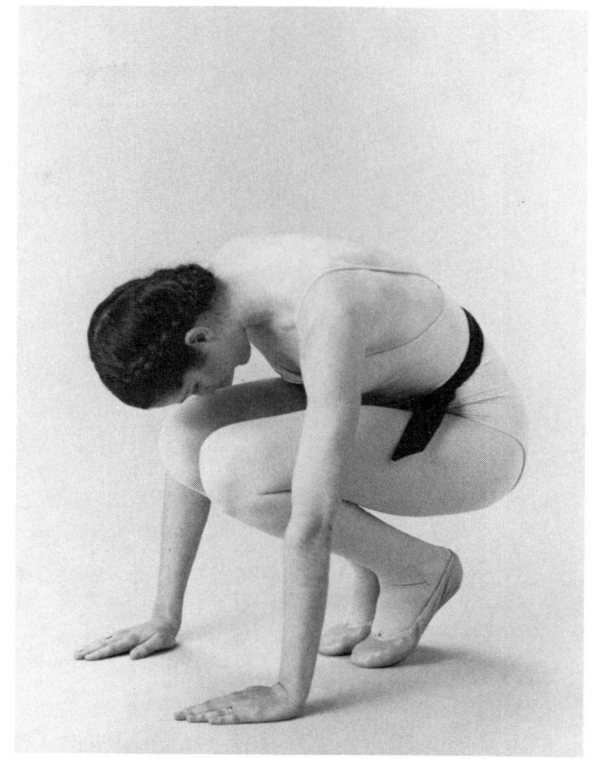

a. *Start a Backward Toe Touch with knees bent.*

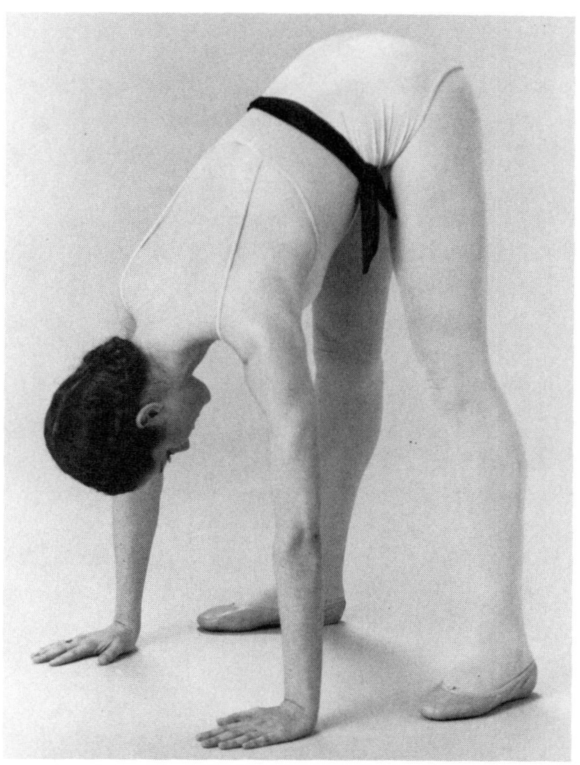

b. *Without moving your hands, try to straighten your legs.*

Ankle Twists

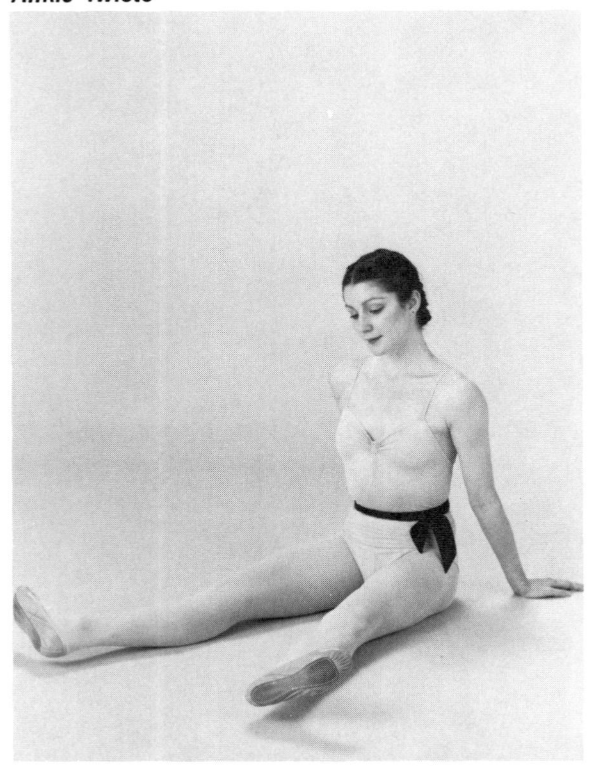

Elevate your legs when you do Ankle Twists.

Toe Flexes

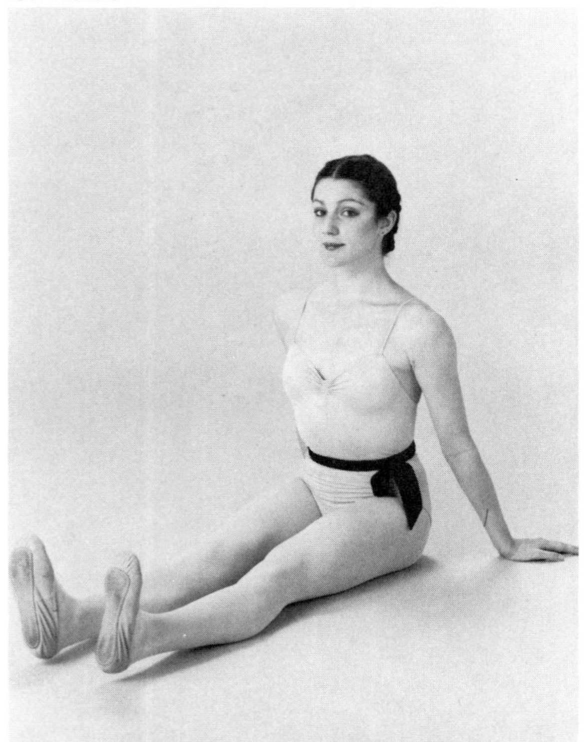

You can do Toe Flexes while reading this book.

Hurdler's Stretch

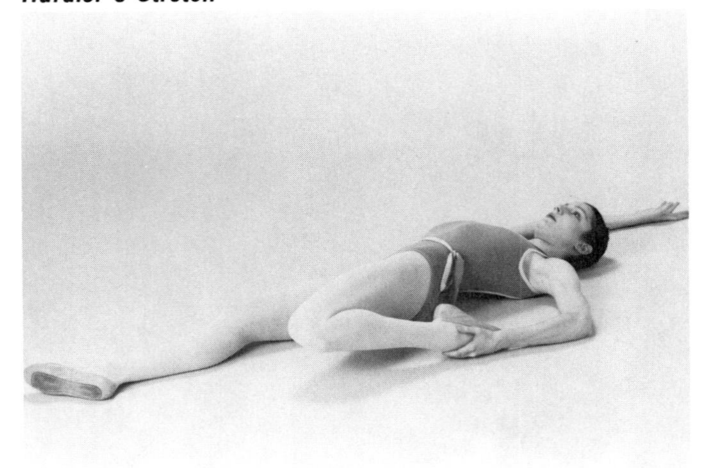

This is a great stretch for the quads.

Ankles

Circles. Sit on the floor with both legs extended in front of you. Put your arms behind you for support. Point and circle each foot around and around clockwise with legs off floor, then repeat the movement counterclockwise. Repeat the movement with the feet flexed. Do twenty. This exercise can be done at your desk, while standing in line or any number of other places. Be creative with your exercising; it's fun!

Toe Flex. Sit on the floor with both legs extend in front of you; alternately flex inward and then point your toes. Do ten.

Quadriceps

Hurdler's Stretch. To stretch the quadriceps, lie on your back with your right leg extended and left leg tucked and bent at the knee. Feel the stretch in your thigh. Hold for thirty seconds, then repeat with the right leg tucked and bent, left leg extended.

Knee Bends. Stand tall. Keep your back straight and your feet parallel a foot apart as you slowly bend, at your knees, into a squat. Be sure to keep the back straight; if you stick your buttocks out, you might strain your back and eliminate any benefit from this exercise. You can do a number of variations:

- Keep your legs close together.
- Spread your legs about shoulder-width apart.
- Spread the legs shoulder-width apart, but this time point the feet out to the side. Do ten.

Knee Bends

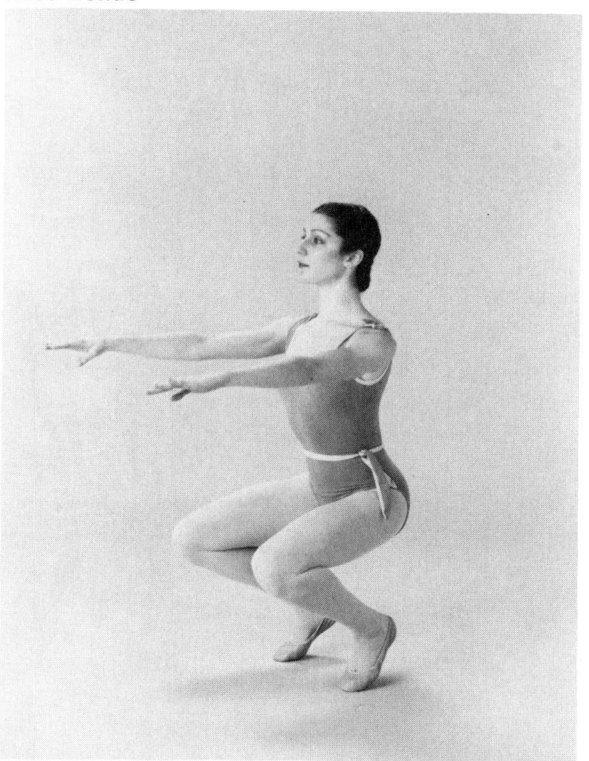

a. *Knee Bends require considerable leg strength.*

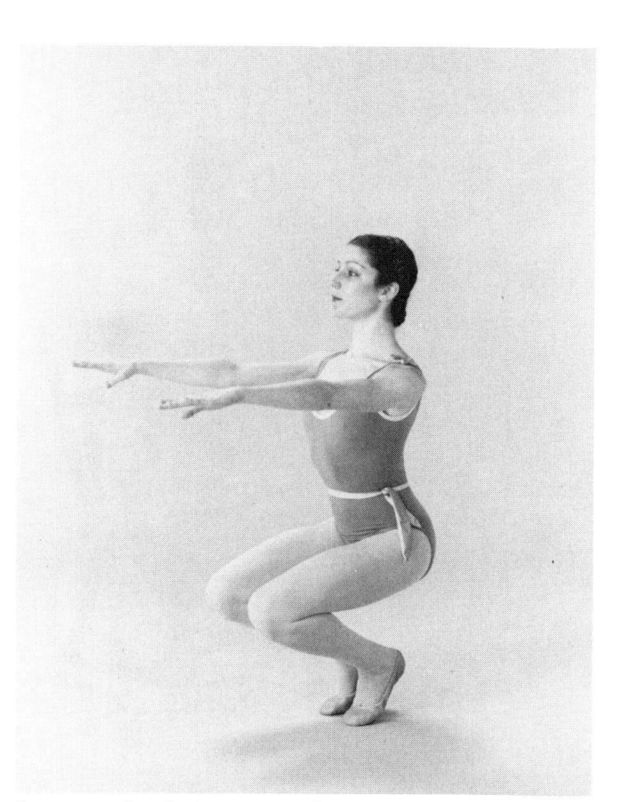

b. *Here the feet are together.*

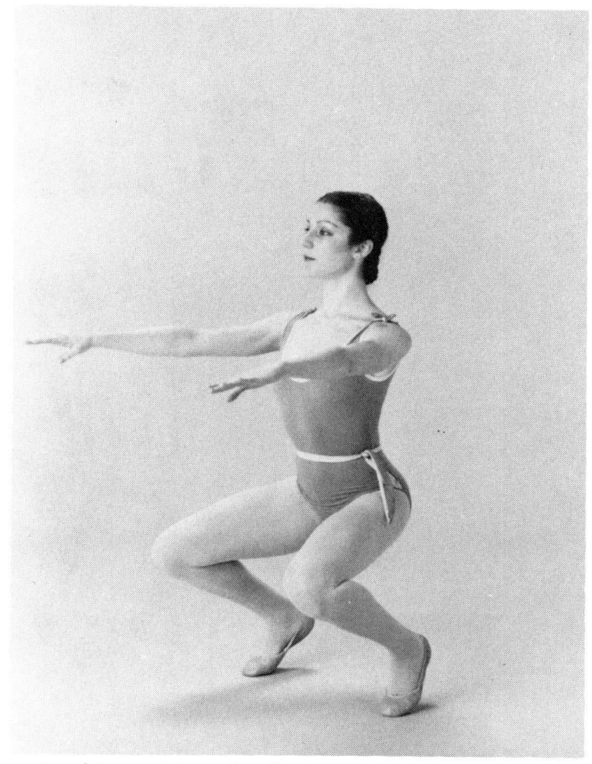

c. *In this position the feet are spread.*

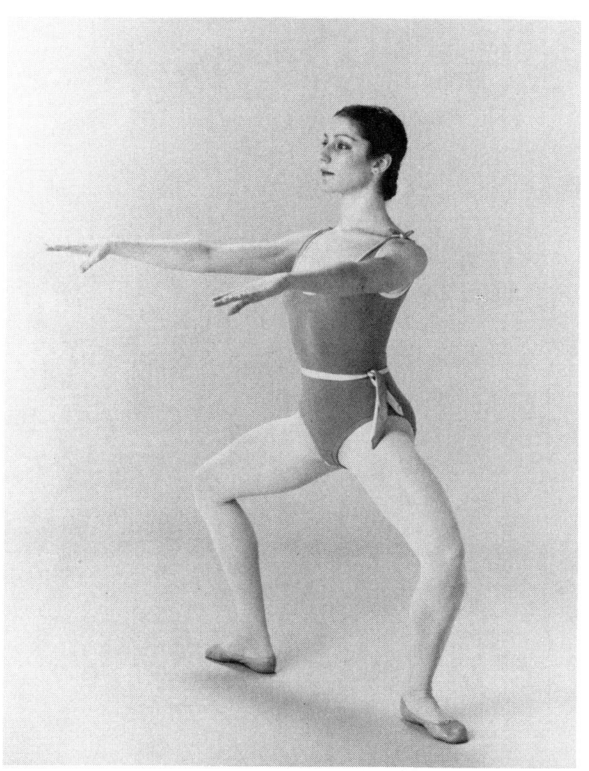

d. *Try Knee Bends with your feet pointed out.*

Quad Killers I

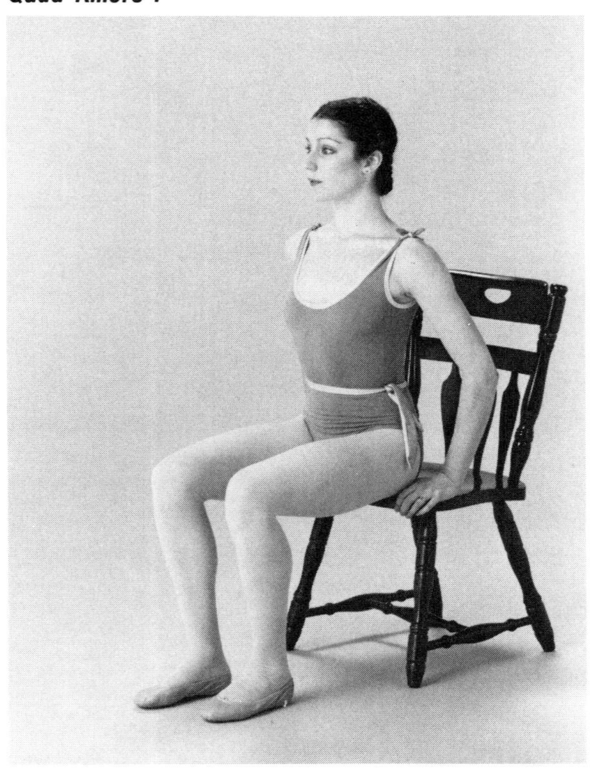

a. *Start Quad Killers I with both feet on the floor.*

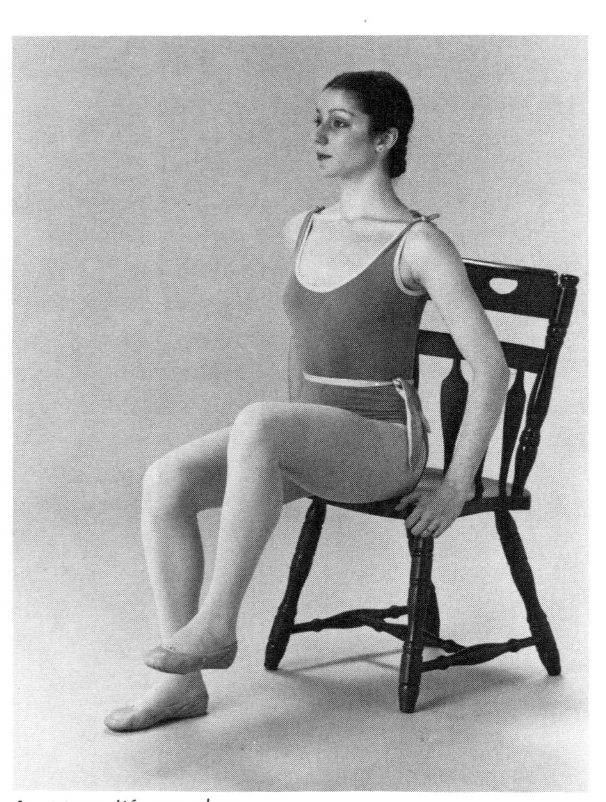

b. *Now lift one leg.*

Quad Killers II

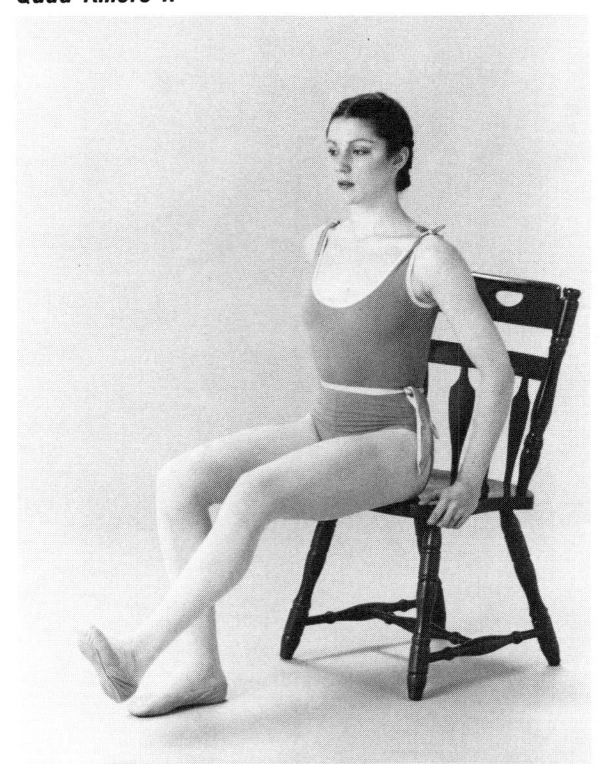

a. *In Quad Killers II you extend your leg.*

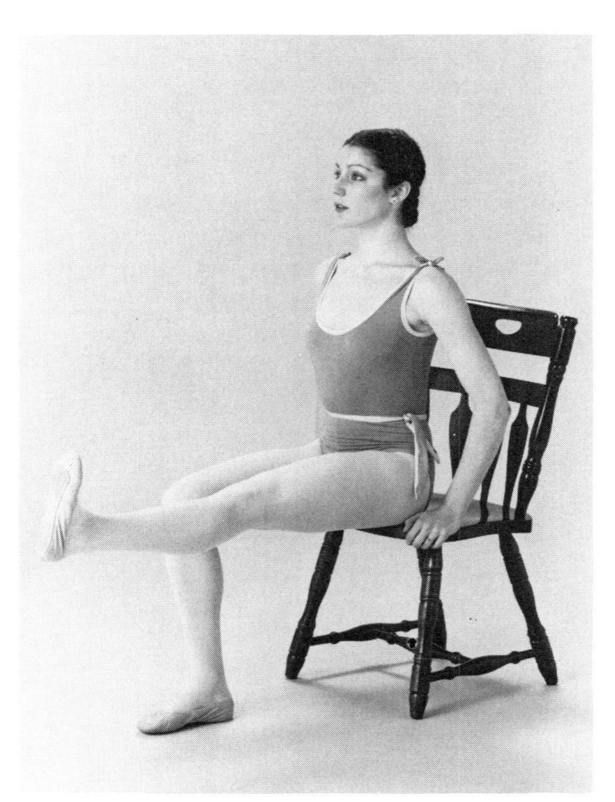

b. *It looks easy, but it isn't.*

Prone Quad Killers

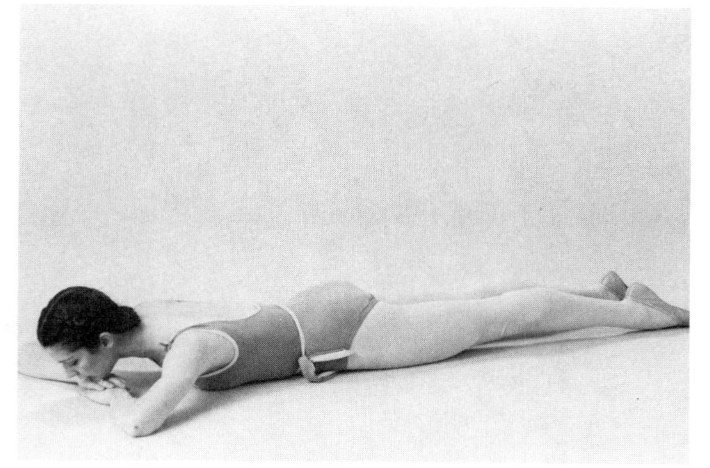

a. *Lie on your stomach to begin Prone Quad Killers.*

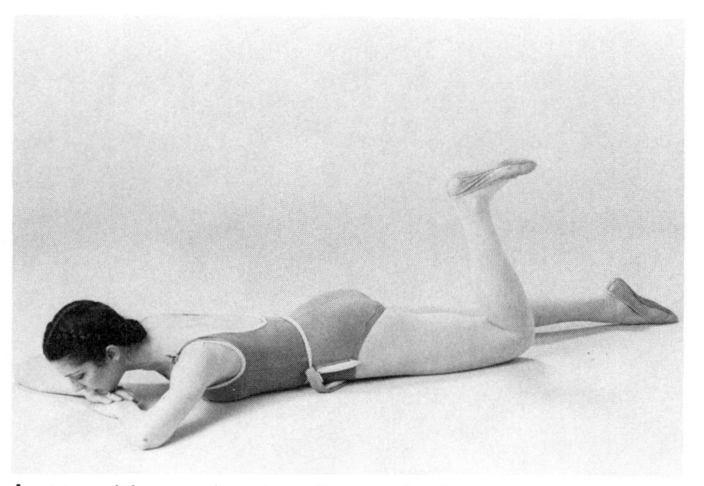

b. *Now lift your leg, bending at the knee.*

Wall Bends. Stand with your back to the wall, feet together. Gently inch your back down the wall as you bend your knees; just before your thighs are perpendicular to the wall, hold the position. Hold for thirty seconds, slowly increasing the amount of time you can perform this exercise. Great for toning the thighs and getting ready for ski season.

Quad Killers I. Sit on the end of a hard chair or bench, lifting the right leg at the hip straight up just a few inches; hold for the count of five, then lower. Do twenty with the right leg, then repeat this movement with the left leg. Strengthens the front of the thigh.

Quad Stretch

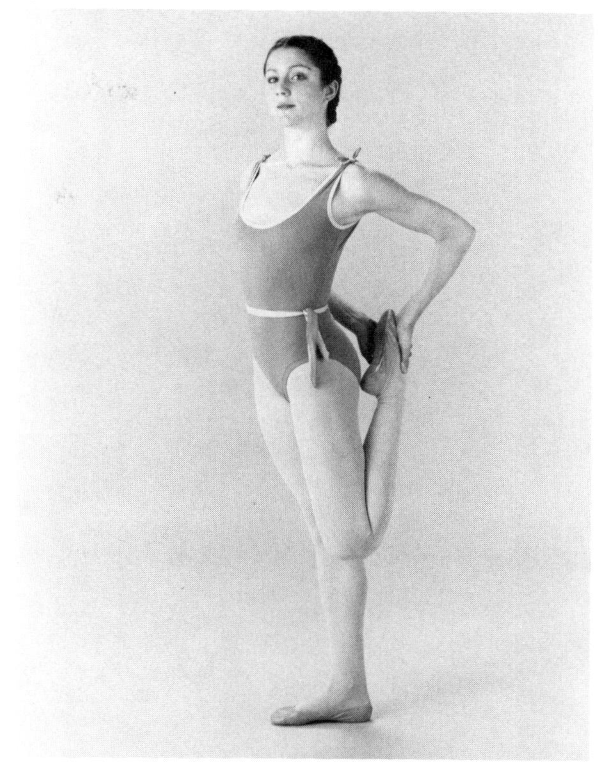

Doing a Quad Stretch is a good way to work on balance.

Quad Killers II. Assume the starting position as with Quad Killers I; this time extend your right leg straight, hold for five, then return to the starting position. Repeat for the left leg. Do twenty.

Prone Quad Killers. Lie on your stomach with your hands supporting your chin. Extend your legs; then, bending the right leg at the knee, pull it straight upwards toward the ceiling. You don't have to move it very far to get the desired effect. This exercise will work your entire upper thigh if you keep the leg strong and tight. Repeat with the left leg. Do twenty.

Quad Stretch. From a standing position, pull one foot up toward your buttock, bending at the knee, and hold it. You'll feel the stretch in the front of the thigh. Hold for thirty seconds, then repeat with the other leg.

Leg Lifts I

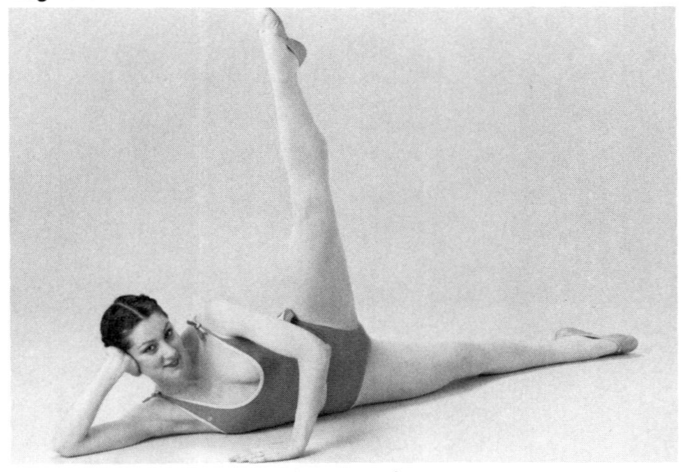

In Leg Lifts I bring your leg straight up.

Leg Lifts II

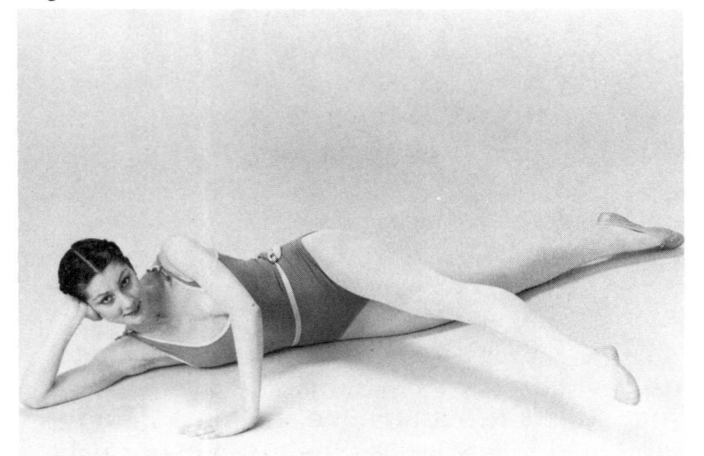

For Leg Lifts II, extend your leg at 90-degree angle before lifting it.

Outer Thigh

Leg Lifts I. Lie on your side with both legs together and extended, one hand supporting your head. Lift the top leg up and then bring it down, keeping the leg straight. Do ten. Hold each lift for fifteen seconds.

Leg Lifts II. Assume the same starting position as for Leg Lifts I, but this time extend the top leg out in front of you to form a right angle with the lower leg. Now lift the top leg straight up. Then roll onto your other side and work the other leg. Do ten. Hold each lift for fifteen seconds.

Leg Lifts III. On your hands and knees, straighten the right leg out to the side and lift and lower ten times. Now work the left leg.

Leg Lifts III

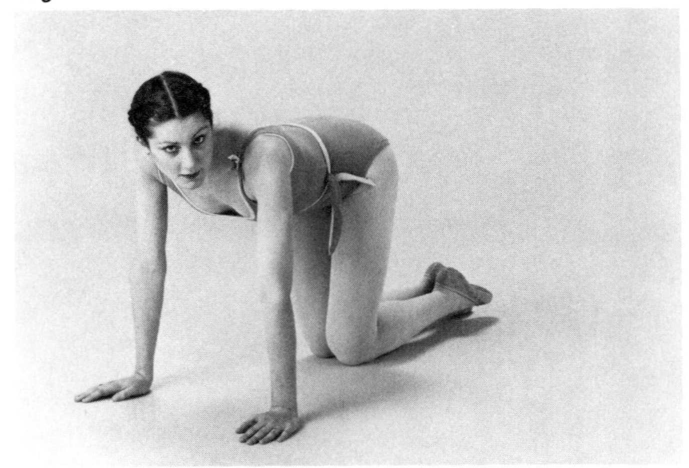

a. *Leg Lifts III calls for being on your hands and knees.*

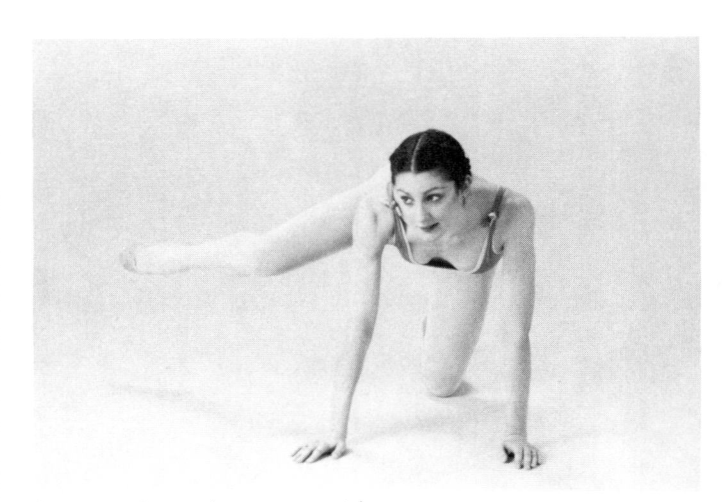

b. *Extend you leg to one side.*

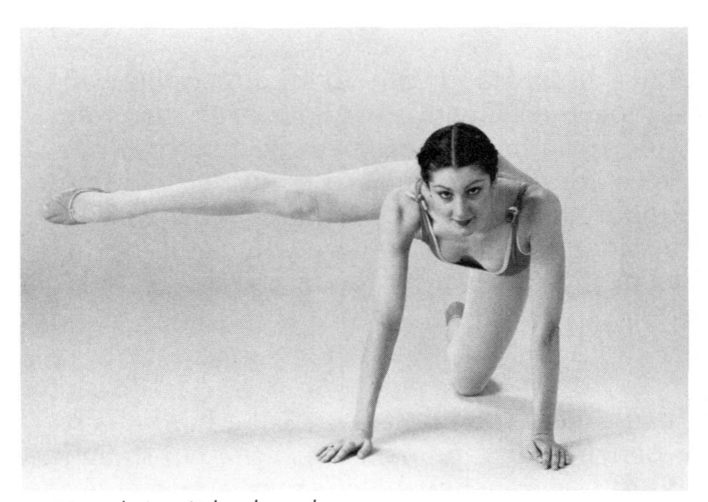

c. *Now bring it back and up.*

Knees In

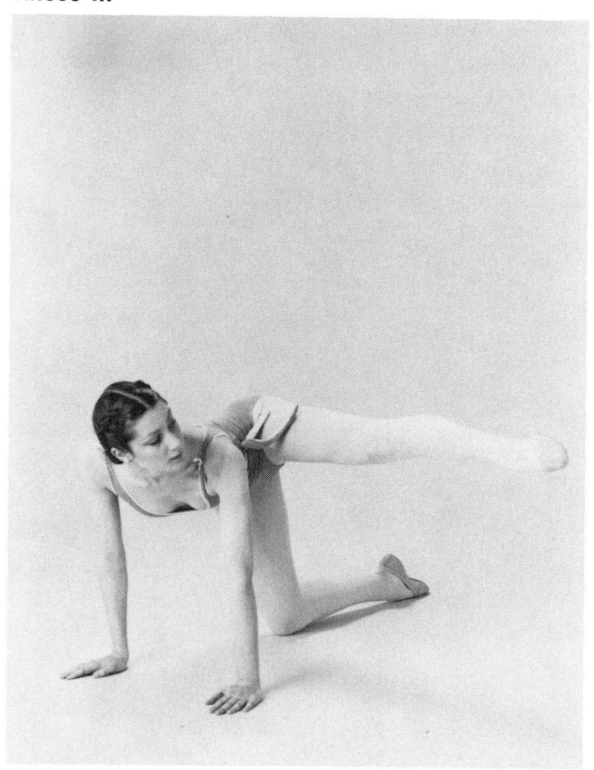

a. *Knees In is similar to Leg Lifts III.*

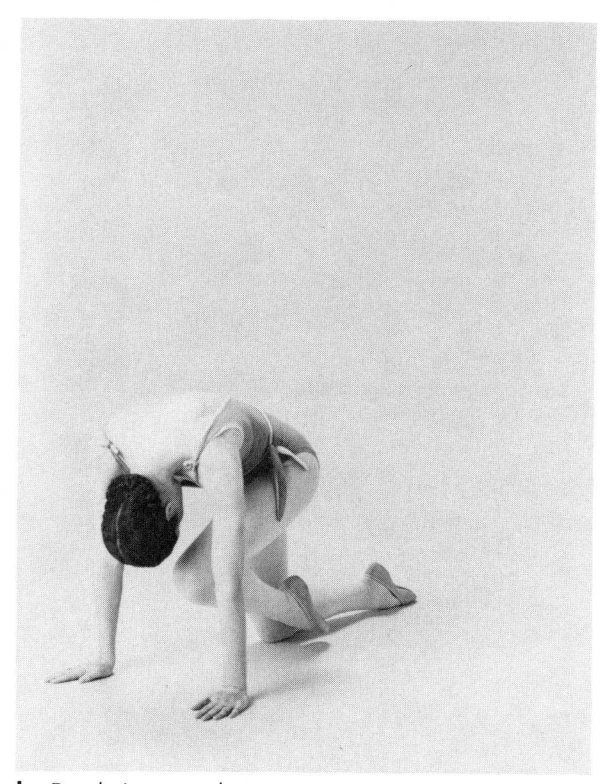

b. *But bring you knee up to your nose.*

Knees In. Assume the starting position in Leg Lifts III, but this time bring your knee to your chest after you extend it out to the side. Bring it in, then out ten times. Repeat with the other leg.

Exercises at the Barre

Everyone knows that ballet dancers have strong, shapely, fat-free legs. They don't just happen; every successful dancer spends long hours at the barre, stretching, assuming positions and seemingly sculpting the shape of her leg. You don't have to be a dancer to enjoy the benefits of working out at the barre. Many women just enjoy the feeling of the luxurious stretches and strength-building positions possible with the support of a ballet barre.

If you don't have access to a ballet barre, you can easily mount one in your home using large-diameter dowel and supports. Another alternative is to use a stool or chair of the appropriate height. Here are five exercises that are commonly done at the barre for stretching the legs.

Long-Leg Stretch. Put your right leg on the barre and bring your body as close to the wall as possible, creating the greatest amount of stretch you can. Now lean forward toward your leg, striving to touch your nose to your knee. Hold the stretch for thirty seconds, but do not bounce. When you feel like you've stretched the right leg completely, carefully bring it down and shake it out gently. Repeat the exercise with your left leg on the barre. Breathe deeply.

Forward Leg Lifts. With your left hand on the barre, standing straight and tall, point your right foot and raise the entire leg from the hip. Keep the leg straight and do not bend the left leg. Repeat ten times, then repeat with the foot flexed. Then do the entire exercise set with the left leg, right hand on the bar. Your body position is important in this exercise — do not allow your back to sway or slump.

Side Leg Lifts. Assume the same body position as you did with the Front Leg Lift; this time, snap the right leg to the side and back to the original position. Point the toe toward the ground and bring the heel back to meet the left heel. Repeat the exercise to the left leg. Do ten.

Long Leg Stretch

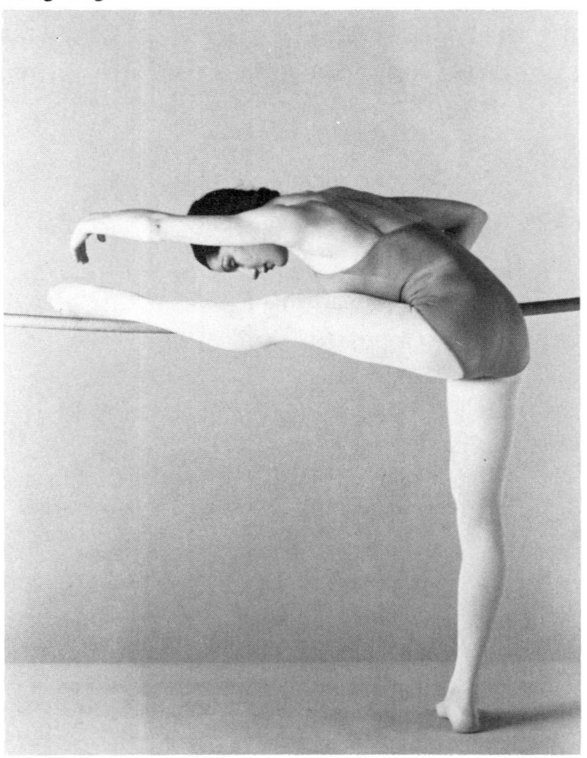

Use a barre for Long Leg Stretch.

Plies

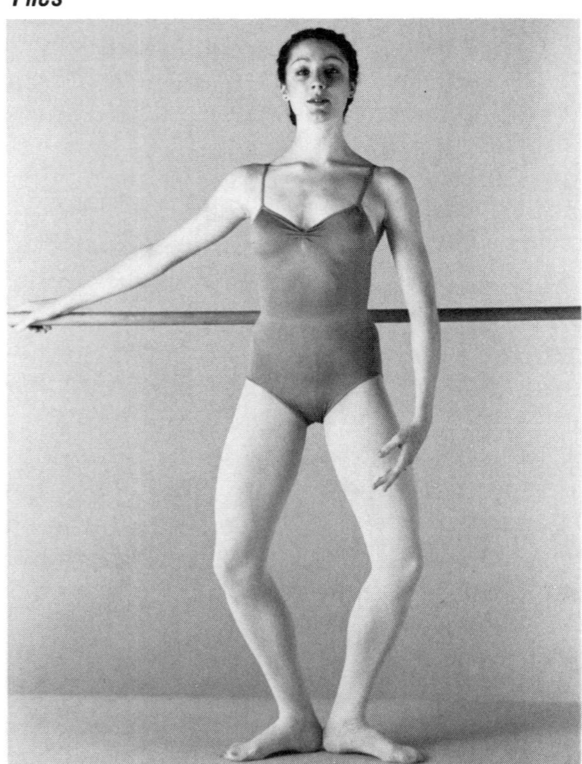

Plies are a required routine for ballet dancers.

Forward Leg Lifts

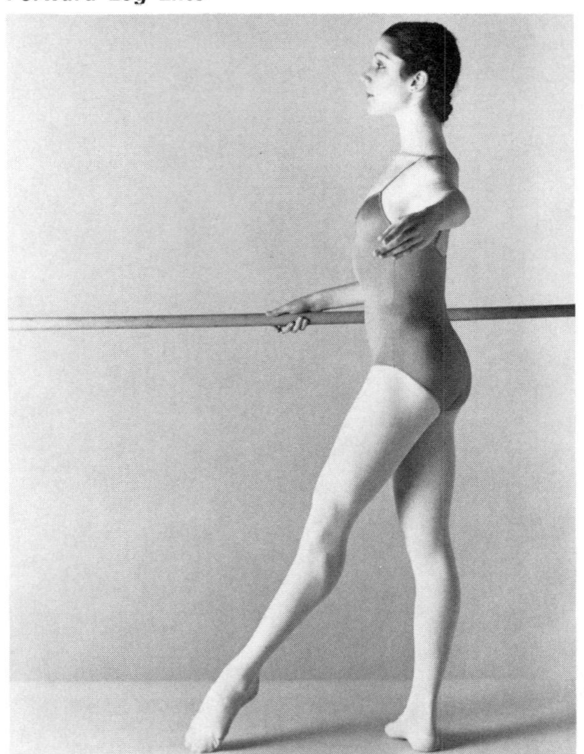

a. *In Forward Leg Lifts stand to one side of the barre.*

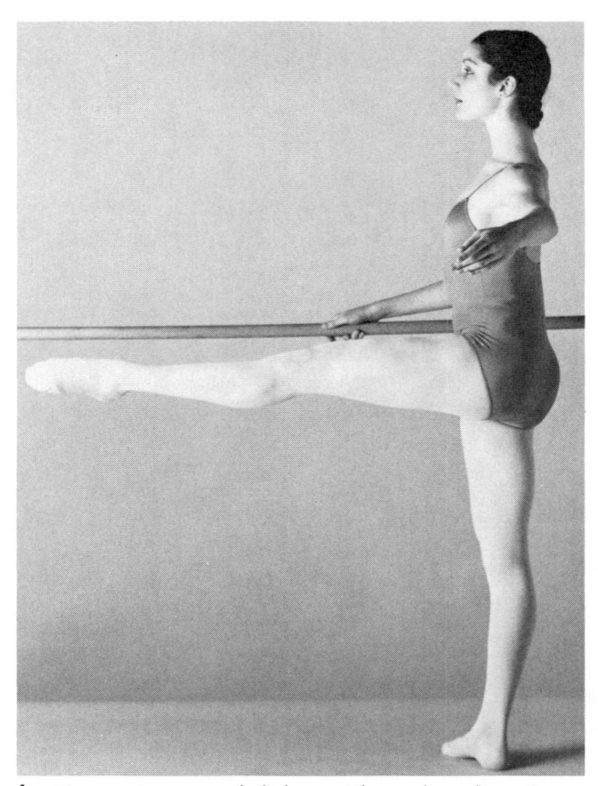

b. *Now raise your left leg without bending it.*

Side Leg Lifts

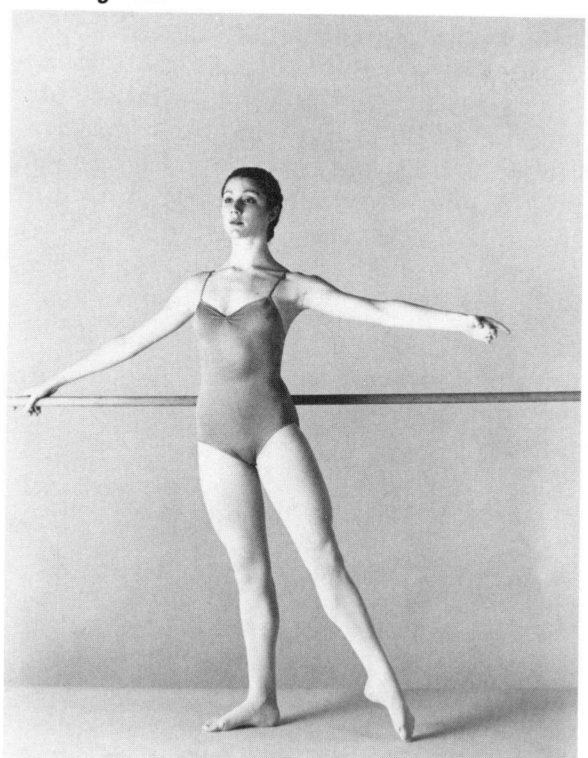

a. *Hold on to the barre with one hand in Side Leg Lifts.*

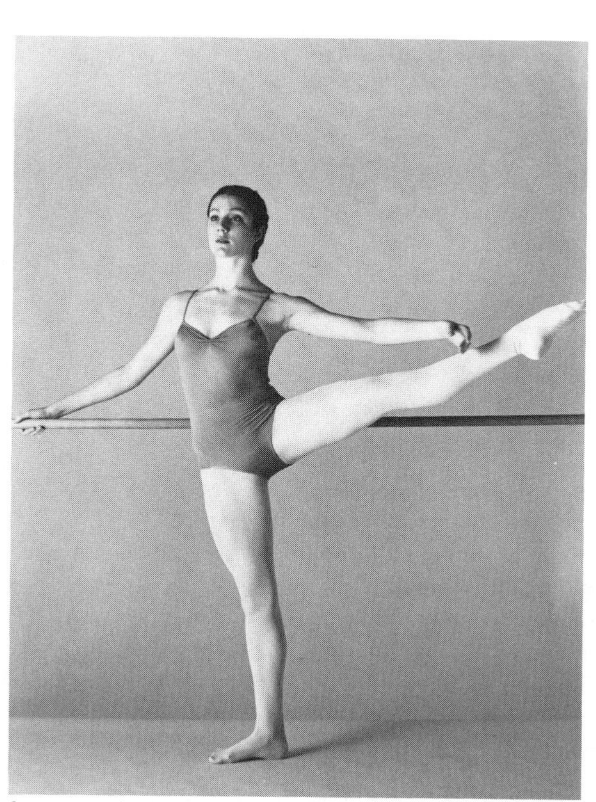

b. *Try to bring one leg up to your extended, free hand.*

Plies and Eleves

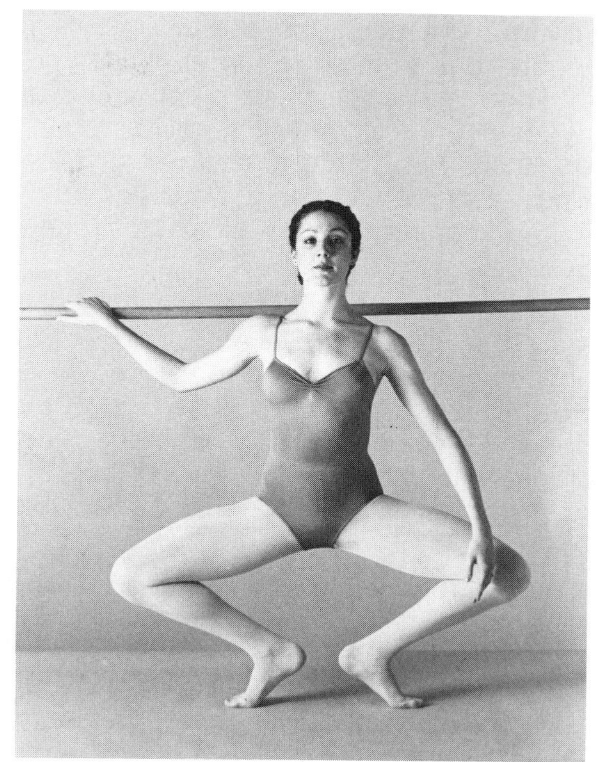

a. *Hold the barre when doing a Grand Plie.*

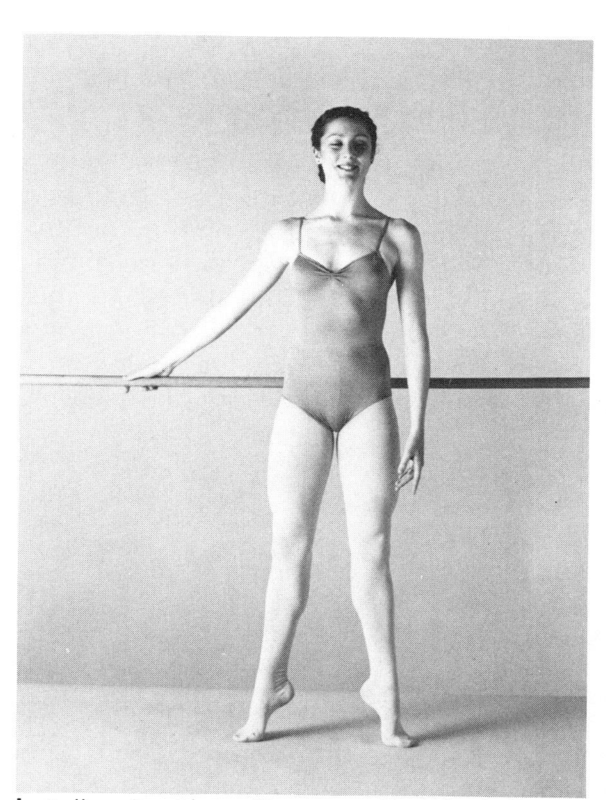

b. *Follow it with an Eleve; stand on the balls of your feet.*

Plies. With your left hand on the barre, stand about arm's distance from the barre, heels together and toes pointed to form a 90-degree angle. Hold your upper body erect while you gently lower yourself, bending only at the knees. Allow your thighs to do the work. Repeat ten times, concentrating on your body position and keeping your muscles taut as they support your weight.

Plies and Eleves. Assume the position for Plies, but this time, after you bend at the knees, gently return to your original position, then come up on your tiptoes. Return to original position and repeat the entire movement ten times. Concentrate on your form and body position.

If you like the feeling of working out at the barre, consider taking an adult ballet class. You may have dreamed of being a ballerina as a child; now you can make your dream come true. Or you may just be interested in gaining poise, balance and flexibility.

TRAINING PROGRAMS FOR YOUR FAVORITE SPORT

Bicycling

Weight training is especially beneficial for the woman who enjoys spending hours on her bicycle. The enjoyment of touring the country and seeing the sights can certainly be diminished if you do not have the strength to keep up with your riding partners. So spend just a few hours a week building your cycling muscles, and you'll more fully enjoy the pleasures of the sport.

Recommended Routine	Sets	Reps
1. Leg extensions	2	10
2. Hamstring curls	3	12
3. Calf raises	1	20
4. Sit-ups	1	50
5. Push-ups	1	25

It's a good idea to do some head rolls, shoulder shrugs and some general warm-up exercises before you hop on your bike. Remember to start out nice and easy, and gradually build both your speed and the distance that you ride.

Running

To be a good long-distance runner, you should be comfortable with being on your feet for long periods of time. Your cardiovascular system should be in top condition and your legs need to be strong. Weight training might improve your performance, and it can't hurt. Since running does very little to increase your upper body strength, it's a good idea to incorporate some arm, waist and stomach exercises in your running workout.

Recommended Routine	Sets	Reps
1. Leg extensions	2	12
2. Hamstring curls	2	10
3. Bent-knee sit-ups (for stomach and hip flexion)	1	25-50
4. Toe raises (to prevent shinsplints)	1	50
5. Calf raises	1	25

6. General stretching before and after every run. The Hurdler's Stretch is particularly good for runners because it loosens the upper quadriceps, which get tight from running.

Your warm-up routine should be gradual. Jog in place for a few minutes or run slowly for a half-mile or so. This way you will reduce your chance of pulling or straining a muscle.

Skiing

Downhill and cross-country skiing require strong muscles, endurance and good reflexes. You especially need strong quadriceps for maximum effectiveness in your downhill skiing. Wind sprints, long-distance running and floor exercises are all recommended. You would rather spend your apres-ski time swapping stories about great accomplishments instead of tales of injuries and pain, right?

Recommended Routine	Sets	Reps
1. Quadriceps strengthening exercises:		
Wall lean	1 min.	3× per day
Leg extensions	2	10
Squats	1	25
2. Leg Curls	1	12
3. Leg Presses	2	15
4. Sit-ups	1	25
5. Upper body exercises to strengthen the arms:		
Arms circles	2	12
Pull-downs	1	12
Arm flings	2	12

9 OTHER WOMEN JUST LIKE YOU

Woman is woman's natural ally

— *Euripedes*

There's an inclination for each of us to think that we're in this all alone; that we're the only one in the world who has a problem with cellulite on the backs of the thighs; the only one who squirms when strolling past the ubiquitous ice cream shop; the only one who hides a pair of "fat pants" in the back of the closet for those days when nothing else feels comfortable; the only one who wonders what to do about hair at the "bikini line." Any of this sound familiar? Well, that tendency to think that we're alone with our physical problems can be very self-defeating, and it doesn't reflect reality. All of us have problems staying in shape; it helps to share both our failures and our successes in order to learn from each other.

In writing this book, I had the pleasure of speaking with a number of women about their regular fitness routines and finding out how they felt about their bodies, particularly their legs and thighs.

The happiest women tended to be the ones that have made a definite commitment to staying (or getting and staying) in shape. They are the women who apply the principle of PRIDE. They recognize that keeping fit is a daily opportunity with exciting new challenges at every fitness level. The most successful of these women see fitness as a real positive in their lives, not as a negative chore that they must somehow "get through."

One of the most fascinating aspects of many of these women, I think, is their willingness to try something that is out of the norm, to be a leader in this regard, and to influence the habits and attitudes of others who are important in their lives. Most have combined their love for fitness with their professional lives, thus creating the kind of lifestyle that many of us only dream about.

Michelle Felsenberg

One of these fitness pathfinders is Michelle Felsenberg of Baltimore. Michelle is a student at Towson State University, and is studying music. A singer who dreams of someday performing on Broadway, Michelle describes herself as "real klutzy as a kid." She began taking dance classes in order to learn to move more gracefully, and she says the results have been positive. "In the summer, I take 1½ hours of ballet classes five times a week. Never have I seen results like that! I love taking ballet, dancing and jazz classes. Sometimes it's hard to take time to exercise, especially with going to school, but it really is important to me. I make it a point to work out every day, even if I'm tired. I know I'll feel better when I'm through, and I always do."

Michelle says she loves to share her fitness commitment with others, and notes, "I'm always showing friends and my two sisters new exercises that I've learned. I'm really careful, though, because I know that I can't push my beliefs on others. But I'm excited because my sisters are considering joining the spa where I work out and teach."

Michelle is one of those rare individuals who has made fitness her pleasure. She's been such a regular at her spa, working out on Universal, Nautilus and floor exercises, that she was asked to join the staff and start teaching classes on her own. She says, "All that exercise hurts at first, but it's the kind of pain that really feels good, because you know you're getting something out of it. I enjoy it, but I know that some people think I'm crazy. However, I know that I don't have any problems with my legs because I'm so active."

Michelle has an interesting outlook on food, and has developed an eating plan that works for her. "Sometimes," she admits, "I pig out like anybody; but on Monday, Tuesday and Wednesday I'm really strict about what I eat. Thursday I let down my guard a little, and I'm strict again on Friday and Saturday. But on Sunday, I permit myself to eat any treat I want. This works for me because I know my body and I know when I start to eat too much. Ice cream and pizza are my real weaknesses!"

Cindy Corralez

You may think that gaining weight can be a disaster for your figure. Not so, assures Cindy Corralez of Lodi, California. Since Cindy began lifting weights, she has gained eight pounds of muscle, particularly in her legs and thighs. She loves the new-found definition in her thighs and calves, stating, "I just can't believe the difference in my body! I've become firm all over and I've even developed biceps that I didn't know I had!" The mother of an active four-year-old, Cindy was especially attracted to the Body Be Fit gym in Lodi because it provides nursery service — a real bonus for this busy wife and mother.

Cindy has also changed her husband's attitudes about her lifting weights as she's changed her body. She says, "At first, my husband couldn't understand why I wanted to lift weights all the time. But now that he sees the great results, he really likes it! He loves the way that I'm so energetic when I get back from working out; sometimes I feel like Supermom and Superwife! Since I've been lifting weights, I don't even mind carrying my own groceries!"

Cathy Lee Dowling

Another woman whose husband is thrilled with the results of her commitment to being fit is Cathy Lee Dowling of Fort Knox, Kentucky. Cathy says that her husband "likes my legs 100 percent now, and he used to call me 'Legs.' " Cathy has been running for years, and discovered that adding weight training has improved her leg structure and the quality of her running. After only six months of weight training, Cathy's 10-K PR (personal record) went from 52:00 to 48:22.

Cathy has found that being fit has helped her in other areas of her life as well. A nurse by profession, she feels more confident about her abilities to keep up with such a physically demanding job. Cathy devotes a substantial amount of time to her fitness program, evenly divided between running and weightlifting.

Lana Edwards

Lana Edwards, twenty-one, of Clifton, Colorado, has learned the hard way, as do many of us. When she started with a Nautilus program, she did not bother to find the amount of weight and repetitions right for her, so she inadvertently began to "bulk up." She added inches to her thighs. She became very discouraged with the new-found weight training program, but under supervision at her club, learned that she should reduce the amount of weight and increase the number of repetitions at each weight station, resulting in a loss of those unwanted inches. And she learned the value of stretching the leg muscles before and after her weightlifting regimen. "I stretch now for twenty minutes before and twenty to thirty minutes after lifting weights," she says. "If I'm really rushed, I'll cut short the stretching to five to ten minutes each, before and after, especially afterwards; that's really important. I also think it's important to warm up on the exercise bicycle before starting to lift weights."

Lana has managed to create a fitness-oriented career for herself. She works at the Nautilus Fitness Center in Grand Junction, Colorado, as an aerobics instructor, and has learned a great deal about the value of regular fitness and exercise. She also knows which exercises work best on the legs. "Calf raises and leg lifts — do them until they burn. You're going to see some results if you do them until they burn, and then push past the burn. Try it, it really works." It worked so well for Lana that she says she can't believe the difference in her calves and the front of her thighs (and neither can her husband). This young woman who keeps photos of Rachel McLish on her refrigerator ("I want to look just like her") knows that what she has developed has taken hard work and commitment and that all that work has many benefits. And what does she say about her strong, slim body and well-defined legs and thighs? "I want more!"

Susan Laughlin

Another woman who has always wanted more and has not been afraid to go after it is thirty-seven-year-old Susan Laughlin. Susan is a free spirit who has all the confidence in the world. And well she should; she has been an Outward Bound instructor and now she owns a new 650 BMW motorcycle. She says, "That motorcycle is the sexiest thing you've ever seen! I'm only 5 feet 4 inches, 111 pounds, yet because I'm so strong, I don't have any problem with the bike." Never one to worry about what other people think, Susan took up weight training in 1978, well before it was a widely popular fitness activity for women to pursue.

Susan swears by the benefits of weight training, combined with a regular program of running and walking. She has found that the only way for her to stay in shape is to get some form of exercise every day, even if it's just walking. What about dieting? "I've tried every diet there is," she admits, "and I've even been on diets and gained weight! I've learned that it's really important for me to eat three meals a day. I just can't stop eating and still continue to exercise; that defeats the purpose of trying to be healthy. It takes a proper balance of good food and good exercise every day." One of Susan's favorite observations about the fitness boom sweeping the country is, "It's wonderful to know that women can sweat and still be respected!"

Celeste Landry

Another woman who has gained the respect of her office coworkers for her commitment to excellence is Celeste Landry of Baton Rouge, Louisiana. Celeste, who has been a secretary for five years, finds that she's considered a "health nut" around the office because she exercises so much and also because she drinks so much water every day. "I drink water," she explains, "because I think it flushes out the system, and it helps me keep from eating between meals." She has noticed that her habits are having a positive effect on her coworkers, as they, too, are drinking much more water and juices, instead of empty, calorie-laden soft drinks.

Celeste's workout routine for her legs includes a session at the ballet barre at least three times a week, aerobic dance and free-weight training. She finds the combination a good one. The program has resulted in Celeste feeling "proud of my body, especially because I work hard at it."

She has learned the secret of moderation in her diet, especially because she loves food. Adhering to the late Adelle Davis' advice, Celeste "breakfasts like a king, luncheons like a prince and has supper like a pauper." Words of wisdom for all. Since this active young woman considers her legs her best feature, she's obviously doing all the right things.

Caroline Smith

Caroline Smith, twenty-three, of Denver, is also doing the right things — and plenty of them, too. She divides her time between teaching aerobics, supervising her house-cleaning business and working on the ski patrol at Copper Mountain every weekend during the winter. That's quite a hectic schedule — and a real inspiration for any woman who says she can't find time to exercise.

Caroline deliberately choreographs aerobic routines to work on specific parts of the leg. Her forty-five minute sessions incorporate fifteen minutes of stretching to complement the intense aerobic workout. She makes sure that the class stays motivated by maintaining a cheerful disposition. "It could be killing me," she admits, "but I never let them know." And her rigorous routines could be killers. She teaches three forty-five-minute classes in a row, three times per week!

This busy young woman who is pursuing her master's degree in exercise physiology is also training for triathlons in her spare time. A veteran of one triathlon in Aspen and two in Denver, she aspires to compete at one in Phoenix and "the Ironman in Hawaii, before I turn thirty."

Susan Lee Soper

Susan Lee Soper of Jackson, New Jersey, didn't want to wait until she was approaching thirty to start taking care of her body. This nineteen-year old college student has been determined to stay in shape ever since she started thinking about it in high school. "I love working out; it really makes me feel good. Instead of feeling fat and sloppy, I feel strong and toned."

Susan Lee's routine consists of weight training, riding the exercise bicycle in the winter and biking outdoors in the summer. Her entire life is fitness-oriented, and she owes a great deal of her interest and success to the influence of her boyfriend, Mike Foley. Mike is a world-renowned diver (he dives off the cliffs in Acapulco) and gymnastics teacher. "Mike sometimes drags me to the club when I don't want to go," Susan Lee admits, "but once I'm there, I am motivated to work hard."

Susan Lee's summer job at Great Adventures Amusement Park also helps her to stay in shape. Not only does she walk at least ten miles each day as she sells balloons to park visitors, but the thoughtful management at Great Adventures has provided an employee weight room. Susan Lee spends so much of her time running around in the summertime that she usually trims fifteen pounds off her already slim 5-foot 11-inch frame. She says that since she has developed an interest in staying in shape she has become more aware of her body, and has "a new outlook on life."

These women that you've just read about are no different than you and me. Each one has personal interests, challenging activities that keep her active and, importantly, fitness goals. Each has discovered, through trial and error, what works best for her own body — both in exercise and diet. They show that juggling our various roles as students, workers, wives, mothers, girlfriends, sisters and daughters need not preclude the scheduling of time to stay in shape. If you don't take care of yourself, no one else, no matter how well-meaning, can do it for you.

CONCLUSION

I know of no more encouraging fact than the unquestionable ability of man to elevate his life by a conscious endeavor.

— Henry David Thoreau

There are no secrets to success in anything that you do. The truths are that you must want your goals — and you must be sure that you know at the outset just what your goals really are. So we can't promise you thinner thighs in three, thirteen or thirty days; we can't promise you slimmer calves by next bikini season. But you can make the promise to yourself. And you can keep your promise, because you made it to the most important person in your life. Don't be shy about wanting the best for yourself. You deserve the best and you know it. So go after it!

BIBLIOGRAPHY

August, Bonnie, with Ellen Count. *Looking Thin.* New York: Rawson, Wade Publishers, 1981.

Bailey, Covert. *Fit or Fat?* Houghton Mifflin Company, 1977.

Brody, Jane. *Jane Brody's Nutrition Book.* New York: W.W. Norton & Company, 1981.

Darden, Ellington, Ph.D. *The Nautilus Book.* Contemporary Books, Inc., 1980.

Delilah Communications, LTD. *Screen Dreams: The Hollywood Pin-Up.* New York: Delilah Communications LTD, 1982.

Edwards, Sally. *Triathlon: A Triple Fitness Sport.* Fleet Feet Press, 1982.

Fixx, James. *The Complete Book of Running.* New York: Random House, 1977.

Fonda, Jane. *Jane Fonda's Workout Book.* New York: Simon and Schuster, 1981.

King, Billie Jean, with Frank Deford. *Billie Jean.* New York: The Viking Press, 1982.

Mirkin, Gabe, M.D. and Marshall Hoffman. *The Sports Medicine Book.* New York: Little, Brown and Co., 1978.

Olinekova, Gayle. *Go For It!* Simon and Schuster, 1982.

Osborn, Susan and Jeffrey Weiss. *The Information Age Sourcebook.* Pantheon Books, 1982.

Paish, Wilf. *Diet in Sport.* West Yorkshire: EP Publishing Limited, 1979.

Paragon Books. *The Decade of Women.* Ms. Foundation For Education and Communications, Inc., 1980.

Partnow, Elaine, ed. *The Quotable Woman: Volume Two.* Los Angeles: Pinnacle Books, Inc., 1977.

Peter, Dr. Lawrence J. *Peter's Quotations Ideas for Our Time.* Bantam Books, 1977.

Rand McNally & Company. *Atlas of the Body.* 1976.

A Ridge Press Book. *The Family of Woman.* New York: Grosset & Dunlap.

Schwarzenegger, Arnold, with Douglas Kent Hall. *Arnold's Bodyshaping For Women.* New York: Simon and Schuster, 1979.

Stehling, Wendy. *Thin Thighs in 30 Days.* Bantam Books, 1982.

Uram, Paul. *The Complete Stretching Book.* Mountain View, Calif.: Anderson World, Inc., 1980.

CREDITS

Models

Augusta Moore, a member of the Corps de Ballet of San Francisco, appears in the floor exercises.
Andrea Klott appears in the weight machine exercises.

Photos

Floor exercise photos are by David Keith.
Weight machine exercise photos are by Rebecca Maliszewski.

Drawings

Drawings by Faye Castelli appear on the following pages: 24, 29, 30, 33, 44
Drawings by Mary Shyne appear on the following page: 26

Acknowledgment

Anderson World Books extends its gratitude to the Palo Alto, California, YMCA for the use of its facilities.